T0122411

DIALYSING FOR LIFE
The Development of the Artificial Kidney

DIALYSING FOR LIFE
The Development of the
Artificial Kidney

By

JACOB van NOORDWIJK

SPRINGER SCIENCE+BUSINESS MEDIA, LLC

A catalogue record for this book is available from the Library of Congress.

ISBN 978-0-7923-6840-3   ISBN 978-94-010-0900-3 (eBook)
DOI 10.1007/978-94-010-0900-3

Adapted from Jacobus van Noordwijk,
De omwenteling die in Kampen begon:
De ontwikkeling van de kunstmatige nier.
Bassum: Nierstichting Nederland, 1998.

Printed on acid-free paper

All Rights Reserved
© 2001 by Springer Science+Business Media New York
Originally published by Kluwer Academic Publishers in 2001
Softcover reprint of the hardcover 1st edition 2001
No part of the material protected by this copyright notice may be reproduced or utilized
in any form or by any means, electronic, mechanical, including photocopying, recording
or by any other information storage and retrieval system, without written permission
from the copyright owners.

CONTENTS

PREFACE

Practical dialysis as a treatment for renal failure began less than sixty years ago, following the availability of cellophane dialysis membranes and heparin for the anticoagulation of blood in the dialysis apparatus. Now at the turn of the century approaching a million individuals world-wide are being maintained alive by this remarkably simple – even crude – 'halfway' technology, the great majority by haemodialysis. How this came to be is a fascinating story, driven by our continuing inability to prevent the progression of the majority of patients with advancing renal failure, or to provide them with grafted kidneys.

Most of us working in the field of nephrology – and many outside it – have some vague idea of how practical dialysis began in several countries at about the same time. But the image of the first practical haemodialysis of actual patients in renal failure, in the Netherlands during the horrors of the Nazi occupation, are already an indelible folk memory. Here we can read about it at first hand, from one of Kolff's associates who was involved from the beginning.

This account is particularly valuable for two reasons. First, because of the detailed background on what happened in the Netherlands during the years of the Nazi occupation and its impact on work with the artificial kidney; and second because it brings to the fore both the mentors and collaborators of Pim Kolff who played – as he himself has always acknowledged – a crucial role in the development of clinical dialysis. Jacob van Noordwijk was one of them himself. Although Kolff himself is of course the centre of this narrative, the team approach that he fostered is evident from this account and has proved invaluable in many countries and on many occasions since.

Finally we learn of the development and dissemination of this knowledge from the end of the Second World War to Canada, the United States and elsewhere, largely fostered by Kolff and other members of his team including Jacob van Noordwijk himself. Beyond that we can follow the technique of dialysis into its context on a world stage.

It is an inspiring story, and an account that will be a valuable source for historians of medicine and nephrology now and in the future

Melmerby   **Stewart Cameron**
Cumbria
October 2000

vii

ACKNOWLEDGEMENT

Mr J. Alexander, the former director of the Netherlands Kidney Foundation, prompted me to consider an English version of the book I wrote in Dutch on the development of the rotating artificial kidney, under a title that was equivalent to 'The revolution that started in Kampen'.

It turned out that many readers, not excluding renal patients living here who dialysed regularly, had had no idea that the technique to which they owed their life had been developed in their own country under the very frugal wartime conditions. That induced me to rewrite this book in English, bearing in mind that this would require adding information that would be common knowledge here but unknown to readers who lived outside the occupied Netherlands in the crucial years.

My brother-in-law Peter van Veen, who had used haemodialysis himself before he received a transplant kidney, again gave me valuable advice on matters that might not be familiar to kidney patients elsewhere.

This book also profits by the valuable advice and illustrations that I received from a number of coworkers of Kolff 'of the first hours', especially from Miss Nannie K.M. de Leeuw, Mrs Mieneke van Dellen–van der Leij and Mrs Willy Arentz–Eskes. The technical information that Dr Walter Zenker collected in his book on the development of extracorporeal dialysis (in German) again served as a valuable background for the present text.

My contact with haemodialysis during the past decades has been a series of views from a distance; I am therefore all the more grateful to Prof. J.S. Cameron for his readiness to write a preface and survey the history of renal dialysis from the viewpoint of a modern clinical expert. In addition he recalled some interesting details of the introduction of home dialysis some forty years ago.

The contacts with Mr Olaf Blaauw representing Kluwer Academic Publishers have been very pleasant, leaving me great freedom in writing this book.

Kolff showed great perseverance and ingenuity in developing the artificial kidney and other artificial organs. I am grateful that he showed the same qualities in helping to save the town hospital in Kampen from demolition: without these qualities the last chapter of this book would have ended quite differently!

The author would like to thank the following contributors of illustrating material:

The Alan Chesney Medical Archives of the Johns Hopkins Medical Institutions, Baltimore – Figure 2.3
Archives University Museum, Groningen – Figures 2.1, 2.4
P. T. McBride – Figures 2.2, 8.5, 11.8, 11.9, 11.10, 11.11, 12.1, 12.2, 12.3, 12.5, 12.6, 12.7, 12.8
Ms W. Arentz-Eskes – Figures 8.1, 9.2
Ms M. van Dellen-van der Leij – Figure 2.5
N. A. Hoenich – Figures 11.6, 12.9
W. J. Kolff – Figures 2.6, 5.1, 5.2, 7.1, 11.7
Ms N. K. M. de Leeuw – Figures 8.3, 11.1, 11.2

Milwaukee Sentinel (November 1949) – Figures 11.4, 11.5

Netherlands Kidney Foundation – Figures 13.1, 14.1
L. Schilder – Figure 7.2

The remaining illustrations were supplied by the author – Figures 1.1, 2.7, 2.8, 3.1, 5.3, 6.1, 6.2, 8.2, 8.4, 9.1, 11.3, 12.4.

INTRODUCTION

The treatment of kidney patients has undergone a radical revolution in the past 50 years. 'Then you just have to start dialysing' has become a common expression for the present generation of grown-ups. It is thanks to Dr W. J. Kolff that this has become a form of therapy just as common as insulin for the diabetic.

This revolution continues to fascinate those who have known the times when the diagnosis of an inflammation of the kidneys implied a death sentence in the long run or the not so long run. Our amazement grows when we draw a mental picture of the circumstances under which this revolution developed. World War II was going on, the Netherlands were occupied and hence uncertainty arose every moment about what was in store for us next. This applied not only to persons, but also to materials. Drugs, bandages, rubber tubing and all other kinds of materials used in medicine became scarce and could not be replaced. The occupying power forced many industries to produce exclusively for the German war effort.

The means to fight bacterial infection remained limited to the group of sulpha drugs, active only against some species of micro-organisms. In addition they themselves could cause dangerous side-effects. One of the most dangerous ones was the blocking of renal tubules by crystals of the excreted sulpha drug. Drugs active against tuberculosis still were only dreamt of. The factotum of the thinking, writing, organizing, creating and playing humans which we now indicate with the letters 'p c' did not even exist in the Utopia described by Aldous Huxley in his novel *Brave New World*.

This revolution in the treatment of renal patients was started by Dr W. J. Kolff in the town hospital 'Engelenbergstichting' in Kampen in 1943. He developed an artificial kidney with a rotating drum that made its revolutions in a bath with rinsing fluid.

Fortunately he gained the support of many persons around him. Mr Th. J. Berk, at that time the director of the Kamper Email Fabrieken (Kampen Enamel Factory) contributed significantly to the design of the first artificial kidney; Mr E. C. van Dijk, working in that factory as a technical constructor, played an important role in the construction. In the hospital especially Sister M. ter Welle and nurses G. J. A. van den Noort and J. H. Raab went for it to make a success of 'the kidney'.

This revolution constitutes a fascinating chapter in the history of medicine and it deserves to be recorded for future generations. To our regret the co-workers of the first hour whose names are mentioned above have all passed away; we can only remember their effort with deep gratitude. The German occupation influenced my life in many ways; one of the good effects was that it gave me an unexpected opportunity to take part in the development of the artificial kidney in Kampen. Although my life afterwards took its course over a different field of medicine my contacts and my friendship with Dr Kolff have remained.

There is a second argument for describing this revolution: the story is not finished yet. The kidney patient must not only be kept alive, but he must also live; that means he must be able to forget that he is a kidney patient. There are organizations in many countries to help the patients and their families to develop a way of life permitting them to take part in the activities they want in the intervals between dialyses; permitting them also to organize dialysis in such a way that they are not limited to staying at home. One of their channels is providing information to kidney patients to improve their understanding of their treatment.

I do hope that reading this history of dialysis will inspire all those involved in the treatment of kidney patients to devote themselves with even more understanding and enthusiasm to the task they took on their shoulders – standing on the shoulders of a medical giant.

Jacob van Noordwijk

THE FIRST DIALYSIS IN 1943

The evening of Wednesday 17 March was like any other one for the few citizens of the town of Kampen who happened to walk past the hospital 'Engelenbergstichting'. They were few in number, for everyone had to be indoors by curfew time and the weather was not inviting. The street lamps gave very little light due to the wartime blackout, and that did not make an evening stroll attractive either.

On the first floor of the hospital, however, any onlooker would have noticed an unusual activity, especially near the consulting room of Dr Kolff. A patient in bed was being wheeled into the room, which was very unusual at that time of day.

Inside the room the chairs had been moved aside. Their place was taken by a low open tank of about 1 metre long in a metal frame, and above that there was a horizontal round metal drum around which a cellophane tube had been wound.

Dr Kolff told the patient, a pale young woman, in a pleasant voice what was going to happen: in a few moments he would draw blood from a vein in her arm and that would circulate through the apparatus to clean it from the substances that are removed by the kidneys in a healthy person. After that the blood would be returned to her vein again.

'Everything ready?' Dr Kolff asked me, as the one who had set up the apparatus. 'Yes, doctor Kolff.' He introduced a needle into one of the patient's arm veins and connected it to a rubber tube leading to the apparatus. Into that tube he injected a dose of heparin solution. The blood was collected into a glass vessel. When about 200 ml had been collected it was siphoned into a rubber tube leading through the hollow axle of the drum on to the cellophane tube around the drum. 'Switch it on, will you.' I switched on the motor, and the drum started to rotate. A soft humming filled the room and mingled with the rustling of water in the tank, that was set in motion by the rotating drum. The colourless fluid in the cellophane tube around the drum became dark red at the end where the blood flowed into it. The blood kept on sinking to the lowest part of the cellophane tube and so that red colour moved on through all the windings of the cellophane tube until the whole outside of the drum looked red. As the blood moved through the cellophane tube the colour became

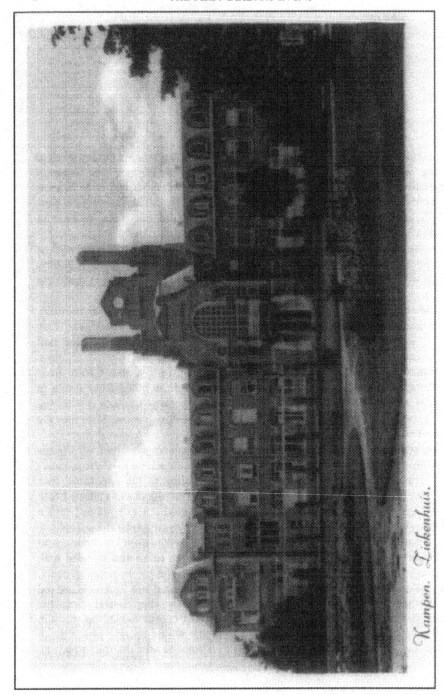

Kampen. Ziekenhuis.

Figure 1.1   The municipal hospital 'Engelenbergstichting' in Kampen, designed by the architect Willem Kromhout, as it was when the first haemodialysis took place on 17 March 1943.

somewhat lighter. The blood left the cellophane tube via a rubber tube through the hollow axle of the drum and then it was returned to the beginning so that it had to follow its way through the cellophane tube again.

After some 20 minutes Dr Kolff decided to stop. The blood was collected again in the glass tube and siphoned back into the patient's vein. At his sign I switched off the motor. The rustling of the water ended; for some moments some water dripped from the drum back into the tank – the rest was silence.

Dr Kolff assured the patient that everything had gone according to plan. He removed the needle from her vein and a nurse returned her to her room after a technician had taken a small sample of blood from the tube connecting the patient to the apparatus. The technician also took a sample from the water in the tank to determine what had in fact passed from the blood into the water in the tank.

The first dialysis was over.

The revolution of the drum had started a revolution that would fundamentally improve the chances of survival of renal patients. It is due to this revolution that chronic renal patients can now stay alive until they can start a new life after a renal transplantation.

2

THE PRELUDE TO THE FIRST DIALYSIS IN 1943

2.1 WHY DR KOLFF WISHED TO DEVELOP AN ARTIFICIAL KIDNEY

Willem Johan Kolff was born in 1911 as the eldest son in a doctor's family. His father, Dr Jaap Kolff, was director of the sanatorium in Beekbergen, just north of Arnhem. While strolling with his son in the neighbourhood be used to make him familiar with the responsibility which he felt as a doctor towards his patients.

As a boy Willem Kolff was so fond of animals that he wanted to go working in the zoo in Amsterdam when he grew up – until his father pointed out that only Amsterdam and Rotterdam had a zoo, and that hence the chance that he would become the director of a zoo would be very small indeed.

His parents offered Willem and his four younger brothers every opportunity for a broad education. He received lessons in carpentry and he enjoyed tinkering, a craft he made excellent use of later on when he started to develop clinical apparatus such as an apparatus for intermittent venous occlusion. He also had the chance to become familiar with foreign languages because his parents made him spend parts of his holidays with families in other countries.

His memories of his secondary-school period tend to arouse very mixed feelings in him. Most subjects he found rather boring – his interest was probably concentrated too much on practical applications. Only after repeating his examinations in three subjects was he able to start studying medicine at the University of Leiden.

After qualifying as a physician in 1937 he wanted to specialize in internal medicine, but then he ran up against a ruling which we find hard to imagine nowadays: neither the University of Leiden nor those elsewhere admitted married physicians to the specialization in internal medicine, probably with the argument that 'a doctor must be available 24 hours a day'. It was only the Clinic of Internal Medicine at the University of Groningen that accepted married doctors for the specialization. Kolff wanted to marry miss Janke Huidekoper – and so they moved to Groningen where he started his specialization under Professor L. Polak Daniels (Figure 2.1). That was a blessing in disguise, for Polak Daniels was interested in the work of his junior

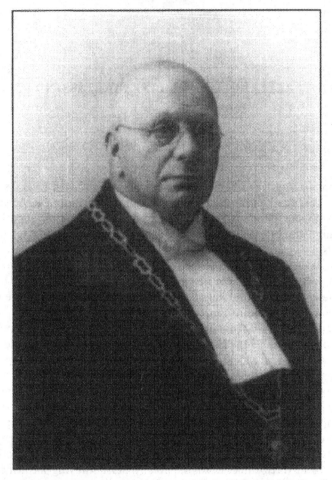

Figure 2.1 Professor Polak Daniels: he was the head of the clinic for internal medicine at the University Hospital in Groningen where Kolff received his training in internal medicine.

assistants and encouraged them – something which did not go without saying anywhere else.[1]

Things were different at the University Hospital of Utrecht, for example. When Professor Heymans van den Bergh was asked there by an assistant to read a paper which he had written he used to respond with something like: 'Sir, so you have secreted a paper? Well, put it in a drawer of your desk and look at it again six months from now – then you will see it with quite different eyes.'[2]

In this period Kolff received for treatment, in one of the four beds allotted to him, a patient who was to give his life a decisive turn. It was a young man who was slowly dying of his chronic nephritis: severe headaches, frequent vomiting, and he slowly became blind. His mother was the daughter of a poor farmer, bent from hard work. When she came to visit her son in her black Sunday gown with white lace cap Kolff had to tell her that the condition of her only son was hopeless. Why 'hopeless' really? Why should a young man have to die only because his kidneys failed? Suppose it were possible to remove say 20 grams of urea daily from the body in another way, wouldn't we be able to combat his nausea and his headache? Suppose we could do this day after day, would not life be possible after all? The young man died.

2.2 THE SEARCH FOR A SERVICEABLE ARTIFICIAL KIDNEY

Kolff delved into the literature. In 1913 three Americans, Abel, Rowntree and Turner, had removed substances from the blood of dogs by making it flow through tubes of collodion that were rinsed in a saline solution.[3] Small molecules in the blood could pass through pores in the wall of the tubes into the saline solution, but the blood albumen molecules were too large and hence remained in the blood. The same applied, of course, for the much larger blood cells. A schematic drawing of the apparatus is shown in Figure 2.2. The passing of small molecules from one fluid into another one, separated by a semipermeable membrane between the two fluids, had been described in 1861 by a Scottish chemist named Thomas Graham. He had used pig bladder or parchment paper, as a semipermeable membrane and he had coined the term 'dialysis' for this mode of movement of small particles from one fluid into the other one.

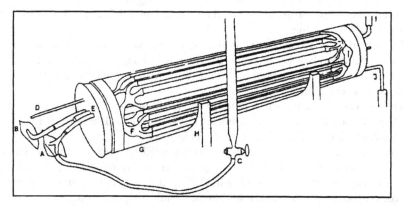

Figure 2.2 The artificial kidney of Abel, Rowntree and Turner (1913) with 16 collodion tubes. A = canula inserted into artery; B = canula inserted into a vein; C = burette with a solution of hirudin; D = thermometer; E = handle; F = flow distributor; G = glass mantle; H = support; I = inflow of rinsing fluid; J = outflow of rinsing fluid. (This redrawing of the figure in the paper of Abel, Rowntree and Turner is taken from P. T. McBride, Genesis of the artificial kidney; however, McBride had indicated the inflow of rinsing fluid with J and the outflow of rinsing fluid with I, deviating from the original figure and from the reproduction of W. J. Kolff's doctoral thesis.)

To prevent the blood from clotting while it flowed through the tubes Abel, Rowntree and Turner had used hirudin, an extract from leeches. Their objective had been to demonstrate that glucose and amino acids could move from the blood into the tissues; they observed that their technique was very effective in removing small molecules from the blood flow. For this process they coined the term 'vividiffusion' and they used the expression 'artificial kidney'.

That sounds very simple, but there were two serious problems: first, they had to mould the collodion tubes (20–50 cm long, with a diameter of 6–8 mm) every time themselves; that implied that they had no standard wall thickness. Secondly, they obtained the leeches from which they extracted the hirudin from Hungary, but that became impossible due to the outbreak of World War I. These three authors never reported on this subject again after their first publication: the reason may have been that the hirudin was no longer available. Abel turned his attention to other fields: he was the first one to crystallize insulin in 1927 (see Figure 2.3).

During World War I the German doctor G. Haas was moved by the large numbers of young wounded soldiers who perished in the field hospitals because their kidneys did not function adequately. He made persistent attempts from 1915 onwards to achieve a 'clinical rinsing of blood', first in dogs and from 1924 onwards in patients.[4] Unfortunately the hirudin extract often caused very severe reactions in patients. From 1928 onwards he therefore used heparin. However, the power of his dialysing apparatus was disappointingly low: he met little support, and after 1928 he gave up.

Another early worker in this field was Necheles.[5] He used tubes made of peritoneal membrane, and he followed Abel's suggestion to compress them between two layers of metal gauze: this resulted in a much more favourable ratio of area to volume.

The introduction of cellophane tubing on the market in the 1920s as artificial sausage skin to replace pig intestine provided a standardized tubing, a marked improvement over the collodion tubing that Abel and Haas had to make themselves every time.

The use of cellophane was picked up by Thalhimer, one of Abel's students: in 1938 he used it to build an 'artificial kidney', so called because it reduced the concentration of nitrogenous products in the blood.[6]

That was the state of affairs when Kolff started to work on this problem. He contacted Professor R. Brinkman, professor of physiological chemistry at the University of Groningen (see Figure 2.4): he had used cellophane membrane for concentrating blood plasma, and he had built dialysing apparatus himself.

At that moment Kolff and Brinkman had at their disposal an effective anticoagulant (heparin) and a dialysing membrane of a constant composition (commercially available cellophane tubing); their task was to design an apparatus with a sufficient capacity for use with patients.

They experimented with several dialysing machines. An aqueous solution of urea was used to test the characteristics of the dialysing machine.

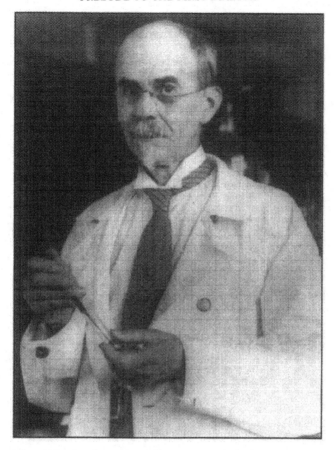

Figure 2.3 John Jacob Abel. He studied pharmacology with Schmiedeberg in Strasbourg and is regarded as 'the father of pharmacology' in America. In 1913 he published the first study on an artificial kidney together with Rowntree and Turner. After insulin had been discovered he was the first to isolate insulin in crystalline form.

In dialysis only molecules close to the semipermeable membrane are able to pass that membrane. To promote this as many particles as possible should be in contact with the membrane, hence the surface of the membrane must be large in relation to the volume of the fluid. Brinkman tried to achieve this by fitting a sheet of cellophane closely over a flat glass plate so that there was little room between the cellophane and the glass. A solution of urea was siphoned in the space between the cellophane and the glass via an opening in the glass plate and siphoned back some time later. This apparatus was satisfactory in the laboratory, but its power was too low for use in patients.

In a second design Brinkman used a cellophane tube into which a closed glass tube of a slightly smaller diameter was introduced in such a way that

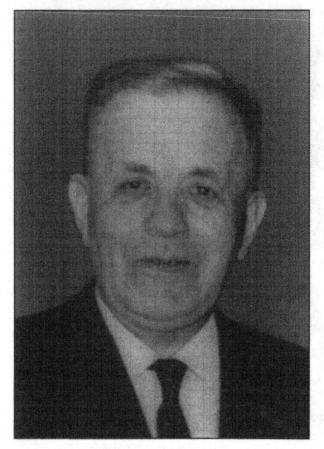

Figure 2.4 Professor Robert Brinkman (1894–1994): the first professor of medical biochemistry in Groningen. His stimulating leadership enabled Kolff to do his first experiments on the dialysis of human blood. He was the promoter of Kolff and of his pupils P. S. M. Kop and E. E. Twiss.

there was only little room left between the cellophane and the glass. By winding a string spirally around the cellophane Brinkman forced the fluid in the narrow space between the cellophane and the glass to follow a long spiral path, providing ample opportunity for small molecules to dialyse into the fluid flowing past the tube. In both these models only one side of the space filled with the urea solution was available for dialysis. To obtain sufficient power for clinical use a 10 m length of cellophane tube would be required.

Brinkman and Kolff finally experimented with another set-up. They took a piece of cellophane tube of about 45 cm, closed one end with a knot and filled it partially with only 25 ml of an aqueous solution of urea, expelled the air from the remainder of the tube and closed that end also with a knot. They then placed the flat sack on a board in a tank of water. An electric motor slowly moved the board up and down so that the water in the tank was in constant motion. The urea solution in the sack originally had a concentration of 4 grams per litre; after half an hour's dialysis they could not recover any urea from the cellophane sack!

Kolff attributed this success to the favourable ratio between the surface and the volume of the cellophane sack; the agitation of the cellophane sack on the board probably also contributed to the effect. In fact the importance of movement for the exchange of molecules through a membrane had been highlighted in Groningen by a colleague of Brinkman, Professor E. H. Hazelhoff: he was the professor of zoology in the Faculty of Natural Sciences and he was interested in the respiration of aquatic animals. He pointed out in his inaugural lecture[7] in 1931 that molecules move very slowly in stagnant water; hence the respiration of aquatic animals always require a flow of the blood and the water on both sides of the epithelium of the respiratory organ. The exchange of molecules through the membrane is most efficient when the fluids on the two sides of the membrane flow in opposite directions. Hazelhoff observed such a counterflow in fish gills. It is interesting that, judging by the illustrations of their apparatus, neither Abel, Rowntree and Turner nor Brinkman seem to have been aware of the importance of this counterflow. Kolff probably sensed the importance of making the water move, for he made the board with the partially filled cellophane tube move up and down in the water. The hollow drum of his first rotating artificial kidney had a fin inside to keep the water in constant motion.

After these preliminary experiments Kolff formulated his objective as follows:[8] to build a dialyser that would move not more than 500 ml of blood continually through at least 10 m of cellophane tubing, and that would make it possible to pass the blood into and out of the dialyser.

One of the models he developed was a vertical drum of stainless steel, placed in a bath filled with a saline solution. Blood flowed through a cellophane tube wound spirally round the drum. A vertical roller covered with sponge rubber rotated around the drum and made the blood move on through the tube. Unfortunately the stainless-steel material required was hard to obtain, and in addition the roller bearings of the drum were affected by the saline solution. Hence work on this model was ended.

2.3 THE MAY DAYS OF 1940

The grandfather of Kolff's wife died at the beginning of May 1940, and so Kolff and his wife went to The Hague on 9 May, leaving their two-year-old son at home. Early in the morning of 10 May they were awakened by the sound of aeroplanes, and from the roof of the apartment where they were staying they saw a German warplane over the city. It was shot down, and the onlookers roared. But Kolff did not attend his wife's grandfather's funeral. Instead he went to the municipal hospital at the Zuidwal and offered his services. The staff expected a desperate shortage of ampoules for blood transfusion: so far these had always been provided by the Red Cross Central Blood Transfusion Service in Amsterdam, but that was out of reach at that moment because of German paratroopers between The Hague and Amsterdam. Kolff offered to set up a blood bank. 'I never submitted a plan which was adopted so rapidly', he declared later. He was given a car driven by a soldier and a second soldier with a rifle (because German snipers were reported to be everywhere) and an authorization to buy anything he thought he needed. Four days later the blood bank was in operation, with a stock of at least 80 ampoules of blood: it was the first blood bank on the continent of Europe. In 1942 the Netherlands Red Cross awarded him the Landsteiner Medal for this remarkable achievement.

On his return to Groningen after the capitulation of the Dutch army on 14 May Kolff also set up a blood bank there, together with the hospital pharmacist Professor T. Huizinga. The importance of removing all traces of pyrogenic remnants of bacteria from rubber tubes and glassware became rooted in his mind, and this gave him much confidence when he developed the artificial kidney.

Kolff was deeply shocked on his return to Groningen when he heard that Professor Polak Daniels and his wife had committed suicide: they had preferred death to the fate they expected to suffer as Jews under a German occupation.

It became clear very soon that the German occupation authorities wanted to appoint a national socialist internist as the head of the medical clinic. Kolff set himself the target of leaving Groningen before this person would appear, and he succeeded.

Some months previously the town council of Kampen had decided to appoint an internist in a full-time position at the town hospital 'De Engelenbergstichting', and in the middle of April the burgomaster of Kampen had interviewed Kolff for this position.[9]

Kampen, a town of about 21 000 inhabitants at the mouth of the IJssel river on the eastern shore of the IJsselmeer, has been important since the 13th century. One of the first towns in the Netherlands to develop a lively trade with the Scandinavian towns on the Baltic it had suffered severely from the sanding up of the river mouth starting in the 16th century. The manufacture of cigars, introduced in the 19th century, brought back some wealth and so Christiaan Engelenberg, the youngest son from an old Kampen family, could leave a legacy to the town in 1910 sufficient for the building of an 80-bed hospital. This was designed by the Dutch architect Willem Kromhout in the 'Jugendstil' style, and it was opened as 'De Engelenbergstichting' in 1916 (see Figure 1.1). For a long time the only full-time position was that of the surgeon-director.

Kolff was the youngest of the seven candidates interviewed for the position of internist in this hospital. His claims were high: a better x-ray apparatus than the one in the hospital in Zwolle (the nearest town, larger than Kampen), a

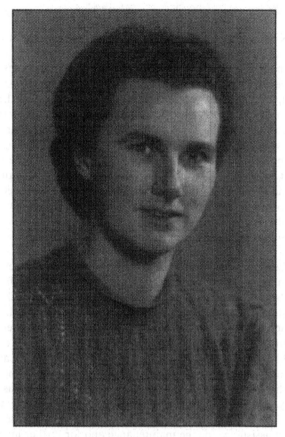

Figure 2.5 Miss A. J. W. van der Leij, the first technician appointed by the hospital in Kampen in 1941 after Kolff's arrival. She was involved right from the start in the experimental work and the applications of the first rotating artificial kidney, in addition to her routine work in the clinical laboratory.

renovation of the clinical laboratory (with the appointment of a technician) and the acquisition of an electrocardiograph were the main ones. He was chosen and appointed as from 1 July 1941. Miss A. J. W. ('Mieneke') van der Leij started working there as a technician in the clinical laboratory; Kolff had met her during her training in Groningen (see Figure 2.5).

In this way Kolff was able to leave Groningen directly after completing his training as an internist, before Dr Kreuzwendedich von dem Borne entered the clinic as the new head, appointed by the German occupation authorities.

2.4   TO KAMPEN: THE ARTIFICIAL KIDNEY BECOMES A REALITY

In Kampen Kolff contacted Mr H. Th. J. Berk, the director of the 'Kamper Email Fabrieken' (the Kampen Enamel Works). He obtained his collaboration for the construction of an artificial kidney with sufficient capacity for treating patients. However, Berk did not see much in Kolff's idea of using a vertical cylinder to support the cellophane tube; he proposed to wind the cellophane tube around a horizontal drum. When the cellophane tube was filled only partially with blood and the drum was rotated, gravity would make the blood sink to the lowest point all the time; hence it would run through the whole cellophane tube. Kolff agreed. This did mean, however, that the blood would have to flow from a stationary tube into the rotating cellophane tube and from there at the end of the drum back into a stationary tube to be returned to the patient. The problem was solved by Kolff after consultation with the local Ford dealer: the system used in the water pump of the T Ford proved to be applicable also in the artificial kidney! Figure 2.6 gives a diagram of the apparatus.

The first discussion with Berk took place at his home in the evening, but it turned out that it would be useful to continue the talks at the factory, where it would be easier to involve the mechanic Mr E. C. van Dijk. That did mean, however, getting up very early: the Kampen Enamel Works had been requisitioned by the German army and hence stood under control of a German official. Fortunately this official never arrived before 8 o'clock, so that Kolff, Berk and Van Dijk could discuss at length from 5 o'clock in the morning on at the factory.

And so it came about that Kolff received his first artificial kidney for clinical use towards the end of 1942: a gift not so much from heaven as from fate – for the factory was allowed to deliver only to the German army and so Berk could not send a bill to Kolff! The apparatus is shown in Figure 2.7.

Kolff needed assistance for the maintenance and for further improvement of the apparatus. So when I asked Professor Brinkman in January 1943 whether

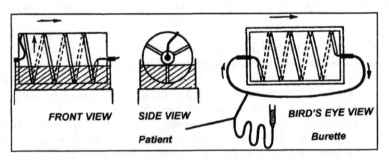

FRONT VIEW   SIDE VIEW   BIRD'S EYE VIEW

Patient   Burette

Figure 2.6   Schematic drawing of the first rotating artificial kidney as it was used in the first series of dialyses. A cellophane tube is wound spirally around a large horizontal cylinder. The blood in the tube sinks to the lowest point. When the tube rotates in the direction of the arrow, the blood will move from left to right. (From W. J. Kolff's doctoral thesis.)

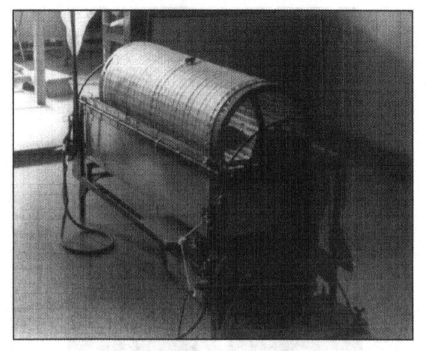

Figure 2.7 The first artificial kidney. The ribbed aluminium cylinder carries 30 windings of the cellophane tube. Blood can flow via a tube visible at the left from a patient's blood vessel via the hollow axle of the cylinder into the cellophane tube, where it distributes itself into a thin layer and sinks to the lowest point. The cylinder revolves and hence the blood moves through all the windings of the cellophane tube. After arrival at the end of the cylinder (at the right in the photograph) the blood leaves the cellophane tube again via the hollow axle. The tube (at the right in the photograph), which has been inserted temporarily into a sterile tube, returns the blood to a blood vessel of the patient.

he could help me find a job for the duration of the war he mentioned as one possibility to start working for Kolff.[10]

In this way I got the chance to take part in the development of the artificial kidney from February 1943 onwards, alternatively as a mechanic and as a clinical technician trainee (Figure 2.8).

At that time the Germans held round-ups of students whom they suspected of anti-German activities. Although I was no longer a student officially (I had been banned from the university because I had been sentenced by the German Supreme Court in the Netherlands for anti-German activities in 1942) I looked like one. One of the general practitioners in Kampen was known to sympathize with national socialism; to avoid his suspicion I exchanged my laboratory coat for a mechanic's blue overalls. Some time later Professor Brinkman obtained an official appointment for me with a Dutch pharmaceutical firm that supplied products to the German army: this saved me from being

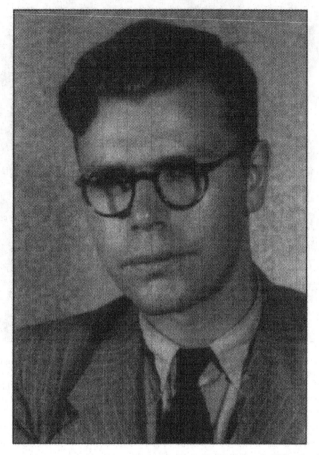

Figure 2.8   The author, when he started work with the artificial kidney in February 1943.

sent to Germany for a long time. However, my personal identity card which, like every other Dutch adult, I had to carry with me during the war, still mentioned 'student' as my profession. Fortunately a bottle of Giemsa stain fell on this document one day and made the text illegible. A dependable civil servant at the town hall took it in without any questions and made out a new identity card for me, stating as my profession 'technician'. Hence I could take off my blue overalls and put on a white laboratory coat again.

When Kolff arrived the hospital did not have a clinical technician. He was convinced that a good laboratory was essential for the good functioning of a specialist in internal medicine. As already stated above, Miss Van der Leij started work as a technician on 1 September 1941. By summer 1943 the workload of the laboratory had grown considerably, also because of the dialyses which had started to take place. Kolff then recruited Miss W. (Willy) Eskes as the second technician. At first he paid her salary out of his own pocket, until it had become clear to the board of governors how valuable this second technician was for the whole hospital. The result was that she entered the service of the hospital on 1 January 1944.

Of course Kolff could devote only a part of his time to the development of the artificial kidney. Although only six out of the 80 beds in the hospital had been allotted to him when he arrived, the demand for treatment by an internist grew so rapidly that he was soon put in charge of 40 beds; that is just as many as the surgeon Dr Kehrer had, who was the director of the hospital.

Kolff received very powerful support from the head nurse of the medical division, Sister M. ter Welle. She urged him on at one time when he hesitated as to whether a patient's condition permitted connecting him with the artificial kidney. 'Go on', she said, 'he has nothing to lose.' She was always willing to change the schedule of the nurses when this was desirable in view of a patient's dialysis. When it had become late at night again after a dialysis she invited the kidney team to an easy chair and a cup of chocolate in her sitting room in the hospital – and that was an extraordinary treat in 1943!

Kolff greatly appreciated her unfailing support, and he showed this by including her name as co-author in the first publications on the artificial kidney.

NOTES

1. The attitude of Professor Polak Daniels was more in line with the opinion expressed some twelve years later by the famous pharmacologist William Feldberg: 'a head of department has only two duties towards his junior staff members: to force them to publish and to keep them from getting depressed'.
2. This was stated in the television programme 'Markant', dedicated to Professor Kolff and broadcast in February 1989. Contact between professors and assistants at the University of Groningen was much less formal than at other universities in the Netherlands in those years.
3. Abel JJ, Rowntree LG, Turner BB. On the removal of diffusible substances from the circulating blood of living animals by dialysis. *Journal of Pharmacology and Experimental Therapy*, 1913–14; 5: 275. Cited by W. J. Kolff, in note 8.
4. Haas G. Die Methodik der Blutauswaschung (Dialysis *in vivo*). *Abderhaldens Handbuch der Biologischen Arbeitsmethoden*, 1935; Abt V, volume 8: 717–755. Cited by Kolff in note 8.
5. Necheles H. Ueber Dialysieren des strömenden Blutes am Lebenden. *Klinische Wochenschrift*, 1923; 2-II: 1257 and 1888. Cited by Kolff in note 8.
6. Thalhimer W, Solandt DY, Best CH. Experimental exchange transfusion using purified heparin. *Lancet*, 1938; II: 554.
7. Hazelhoff EH. Air and water as the environment for animal life (In Dutch). Inaugural lecture as Professor of Zoology at the University of Groningen, 1931. He died unexpectedly in the summer of 1945. He was particularly interested in the exchange of gases and solutes between the blood of animals and their environmental (water or air) and it would have been interesting to hear his comments when Kolff obtained his doctorate in January 1946!
8. W. J. Kolff. De kunstmatige nier (The artificial kidney). Thesis for the Doctorate in Medicine at the University of Groningen on 16 January 1946. Kampen: J. H. Kok NV.
9. Van Mierlo R. Van liefdadigheid tot moderne gezondheidszorg: 75 jaar Stadsziekenhuis Engelenbergstichting in Kampen (From charity to modern health care: 75 years Municipal Hospital Engelenbergstichting in Kampen). Kampen: J. H. Kok, 1991.
10. How I came to work with Kolff. I had started studying medicine in Groningen in 1938 and I

would have done my 'candidaats' examination in the summer of 1941 (rounding off the stage devoted mainly to normal man) if I had not been arrested in March 1941 by the Gestapo for being active for the underground student periodical *De Geus onder studenten* ('The Geus among students', Geus being the classical Dutch name for freedom fighters in the 80 years war of independence 1568–1648).

After 11 months detention in the police prison in Scheveningen I was brought before the 'Deutsches Obergericht in den besetzten niederländischen Gebieten' (German Supreme Court in the occupied Dutch territories) with 64 others. I was sentenced to 18 months imprisonment. When I was set free on 16 September 1942 my name was one on the list of approximately 10 students who were no longer allowed to be enrolled as students because of their anti-German conduct. Curiously enough this did not exclude me from doing university examinations. I studied at home and passed my 'candidates' examination in January 1943, that is before students in the Netherlands had to sign a declaration of loyalty to the German authorities in order to be allowed to study at a university.

Of course I was convinced (like most people in the Netherlands) that Germany would lose the war so that I would be able to finish my studies after all, but I did have to find some kind of work while the war lasted.

In fact Professor Brinkman informed me of two possibilities. He knew that Kolff needed some help and he knew also that the pathologist of the Canisius hospital in Nijmegen needed someone to help with autopsies. The advantage would be that I would be able to declare that I had been present at 200 autopsies, as required for doing the next medical examination, when I would resume my studies after the end of the war.

I visited both Kolff in Kampen and the pathologist in Nijmegen. On the way back from Nijmegen by train I decided to accept the job in Nijmegen; I had caused a lot of trouble to my parents by my imprisonment and I felt a moral duty to finish my studies after the war as rapidly as possible. Hence I wrote a letter to Kolff thanking him again for the way he had received me in Kampen, but I also told him that I had decided to go to Nijmegen, for the reason given above.

That evening I regretted that letter deeply. Was it really so important to add another physician to the enormous number there already? If I went to Nijmegen, yes; there would be one more most rapidly – but if I went to Kampen I might perhaps assist in the development of a completely new possibility in medicine.

The house where I had a room had no telephone, but at the corner of the street there was a shop that did have one. As soon as it opened I went there and I phoned Kolff. I told him I had written him a letter with my decision to prefer Nijmegen, but I asked him whether I could come back on that. 'Yes, provided you do it damn quickly' was his reaction. 'Can I start work with you on Monday?' I asked. 'Yes' was his answer.

And so my work in Kampen started on Monday 8 February 1943.

3

STEP BY STEP TOWARDS A ROBUST MACHINE

On the morning after the first dialysis the patient said she felt much better. That must have been due to the hope the whole procedure had given her, for the total quantity of substance which had passed from her blood into the rinsing fluid was too small to explain this effect.

The first dialysis had shown that a patient can tolerate such a procedure quite well, and that was an encouragement to go on. It encouraged Kolff to make the following dialyses longer and longer. Very soon the habit grew in the hospital to say 'the kidney' when the artificial kidney was meant; that will also be done from now on in this text unless of course a natural kidney is meant.

Kolff initially wanted to develop a kidney that would stand by ready for use so that it could be switched on at any moment. That implied that all parts through which blood would flow had to constitute a sterile closed circuit.

At Kolff's suggestion I tried to sterilize the blood circuit of the kidney by perfusing it with a 0.1% solution of oxyquinoline sulphate; however, this was not sufficient to kill all bacteria. Neither did variants of this technique enable us to prevent any bacterial infection of the blood circuit. Later we tried to mount-sterilize all parts of the circuit, put them together aseptically and keep the blood circuit sterile by filling it with alcohol. Unfortunately the cellophane tube became brittle when it dried on the outside, shrank and cracked, causing leaks. We tried to prevent this by applying glycerine on the outside, the technique the cellophane manufacturer used to keep it supple. Unfortunately a surplus of glycerine damaged the erythrocytes. The best solution proved to be to sterilize all parts of the blood circuit immediately before use, and assemble them.

3.1 TOWARDS A CONTINUOUS PERFUSION

The effect of a dialysis was determined from the change in the patient's blood urea concentration and from the mass of urea recovered from the rinsing fluid.

In the first six dialyses about half a litre of blood flowed several times through the cellophane tube before being returned to the patient's vein. The blood urea concentration fell markedly during this circulation through the kidney, but the total amount of urea that was removed per hour was low. It was not until the fifth dialysis that we found a slight lowering of the blood urea level of the patient: more than 4 litres of blood flowed through the artificial kidney and about 13 grams of urea were washed out.

Kolff expected that the yield of the dialysis would increase if the blood flowed through the kidney continuously, and no longer in small portions circulating through the kidney several times before being returned to the patient. Hence he changed over to continuous perfusion in the seventh dialysis. The expectation was that the blood would collect more urea and other waste products from the tissues.

He injected a needle into the patient's femoral artery through the skin of the groin and returned the blood after perfusion of the kidney via a needle in a vein. Everything went fine until the arterial needle was retracted from the artery after the dialysis. The wound continued to bleed in spite of the tourniquet that usually stops an arterial haemorrhage. Only when the patient was brought to the operating table to enable the surgeon to suture the artery did the bleeding stop. Continuous perfusion was made possible in the eighth and ninth dialyses by exposing one of the patient's arteries and introducing into it a wide needle to carry the blood to the kidney. A glass cannula was introduced into an exposed artery in subsequent dialyses, instead of a needle.

In the tenth dialysis blood was taken from the patient via a needle introduced into a vein, and returned via a needle in another vein. In this way 18 litres of blood flowed through the kidney in 6 hours, i.e. about three times the total blood volume of about 5 litres. We reached a yield of 35 grams of urea.

A radial artery was exposed for the eleventh dialysis and a needle was introduced in it. Unfortunately the blood did not flow well from this artery, and the dialysis had to be terminated rapidly. This artery kept on bleeding for 3 days. The twelfth dialysis was also a failure: a leak appeared in the radial artery, and Kolff decided to give up the operation.

Continuous perfusion was used in all subsequent patients. At first the blood was taken from a vein, but later an artery was exposed so that a glass cannula could be introduced to bring the blood to the kidney.

At first a burette was used to collect the blood for returning it to the patient; from the burette it was siphoned into the return tube. To return the blood rapidly we hoisted the burette up to the ceiling of the room with a pulley. The drawback was that it was hard to see whether the burette was almost empty. Fortunately I had a pair of opera glasses to monitor this return flow. Later we used a roller tube pump to return the blood to the patient: the advantage was that the blood flow from and to the patient was more uniform. Figure 3.1 shows the path of the blood through the dialyser from then on.

3.2 THE YIELD OF THE DIALYSIS

After Kolff had proceeded to a continuous perfusion of the artificial kidney the total amount of urea recovered from the rinsing fluid increased. However,

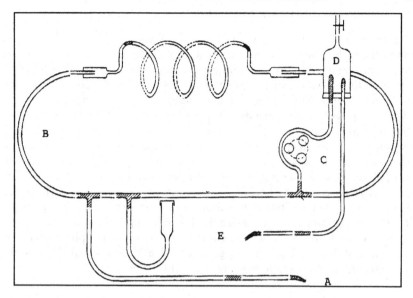

Figure 3.1 Diagram of the rotating artificial kidney as it was used for continuous blood flow. Blood from an artery enters the cellophane tube via (A) and (B). After flowing though the cellophane tube the blood is returned to a vein by a roller pump (C) via an air trap (D). Glass cannulae and joints are shaded.

the treatment lasted much longer than in the first series of six dialyses. Table 3.1 shows the yield per hour from the fractionated dialyses and from the continuous dialyses in which blood flowed either from an artery or from a vein. These figures support the hypothesis that continuous perfusion has a higher yield than a fractionated one. As a matter of fact we must be cautious in comparing the yields of continuous perfusion; several other factors also play a role, such as the blood urea level at the beginning of the dialysis. Hence these figures should not induce us to attach any weight to the difference in yield between taking blood from an artery and taking it from a vein.

Table 3.1 The yield of different types of dialysis

		Grams of urea removed	
Type of dialysis	Number	Per hour	Per litre of blood
Small fractions	6	2.45	2.38
Continuous from an artery	15	9.17	1.69
Continuous from a vein	6	7.85	2.69

3.3   PROTECTION OF ERYTHROCYTES DURING DIALYSIS

It struck us that the blood collected from the kidney after the sixth dialysis showed haemolysis after standing for a day. We suspected this to be due to mechanical damage because we compressed the cellophane tube by hand to empty it at the end of the dialysis, and in doing so our hands repeatedly struck the ribs of the drum. Rinsing the cellophane tube with the oxyquinoline solution had no effect. Kolff then remembered that glucose was added to the blood in a blood bank to improve its conservation. Hence he used a rinsing fluid containing 1.5% of glucose and 0.7% of sodium chloride in the subsequent dialyses, instead of a mixture of salts resembling as far as possible the composition of blood plasma after removal of the plasma proteins. From that time on we no longer observed any haemolysis. Only when the dialyses started to last much longer, so that 80 litres of blood or more flowed through the apparatus, did it prove necessary to use a rinsing fluid with a composition that was more closely adapted to the needs of the patient. We were of the opinion that the replacement of sharp steel needles by glass cannulae without sharp edges would also contribute to reducing damage to the erythrocytes.

4

IN THE MEANTIME THE WAR WENT ON

It is probably very hard for the reader who has no personal experience of life during World War II under the German occupation to get a clear picture of the circumstances under which Kolff led this development.

Food shortage plays a dominant role in stories about the war in Holland, but this applies mainly to the situation in the provinces of North and South Holland from the autumn of 1944 until the end of the war in May 1945. From 1940 on the food supply was restricted and food was monotonous, without much luxury, but certainly in the eastern part of the country most people were able to obtain enough energy from their food, either through the rationing system, producing their own food, or through a grey or black market. This certainly applied to Kampen, where a number of people managed, for example to obtain milk from farmers in the neighbourhood without rationing coupons.

The mental problems were much more severe. Although only a limited number of Dutch people sympathized with national socialism, we had to learn to be extremely careful about what we said in public. Telephone lines could be tapped; hence they were not to be used for anything but strictly personal matters. Radio sets had to be handed in to the German authorities in the course of 1942; that meant that news of the war from allied broadcasts could be received only by those who had managed to keep a radio set hidden somewhere. All this was at least a decade before the development of the transistor: all radio sets used valves, consuming much more power than the transistors nowadays. Hence there were no hand-held portable radios, that are easy to hide, but only radio sets that obtained their power from the mains or from large bulky batteries – not so easy to carry around.

We had to be careful to whom we told such radio news – being found out by the German authorities could mean imprisonment and death, especially towards the end of the war. Life became extremely unpredictable: we never knew what new decree would be published by the German authorities, what new threat lay ahead of us.

In 1943 the German authorities decreed that all medical doctors had to become members of the 'Artsenkamer' (Physicians Chamber) as in Nazi Germany. A large majority of doctors refused. They sent a letter of protest to the German Reichskommissar for the Occupied Territories and they covered

23

the title 'arts' ('medical doctor') on their name-plate with sticking plaster.
Fortunately these letters arrived at the Reichskommissars's office in such enormous numbers that taking measures against all the senders was clearly impossible. However, one of the general practitioners in Kampen, a very precise man,
had prepared the letter in advance and put it on the mantelpiece, ready for
mailing. When his son came home from school that day he saw the letter and,
wishing to please his father, he posted it the same day. The result was that the
Reichskommissar received one letter from one doctor: he was arrested immediately and sent to the concentration camp near Amersfoort. Fortunately he was
released when it became apparent that he was just one of the hundreds of
doctors who sent such a letter.

One day in 1943 Kolff said to me 'I expect there will be trouble shortly;
you'd better go away for some days.' Of course I did not ask why: it had
become second nature not to react with questions to such warnings, for if you
did not know anything you could not be forced to confess it if you were
arrested by the Germans. I left Kampen and stayed some days with the parents
of one of my friends. He had gone underground because he refused to sign the
declaration of allegiance to the German authorities, which all university students were compelled to sign in order to go on with their studies.

After a few days away from Kampen I inquired carefully how things were
in Kampen. Kolff said I could come back. Only decades after the war Kolff
told me why he had warned me. The underground resistance movement had
made plans to shoot the Nazi head of police of Kampen the moment his car
emerged from the old town gate to drive along the quay of the IJssel river. A
member of the resistance movement would stand there with an easel, pretending
to be engaged in sketching the medieval gate. As soon as he had shot the head
of police he would be taken outside the town in Kolff's car, to allow him to
escape as quickly as possible. However, that day the car of the head of police
was accompanied by another car – and the resistance man felt that the chance
of getting away after shooting the head of police would be minimal – so he
did not shoot, but made his way as quickly and unobtrusively as he could. He
ran to Kolff to take him out of town as rapidly as possible. Nothing happened
that time.

In September 1944 the German occupation authorities compelled men in
Kampen to build trenches to delay the advance of the allied troops; Kolff
advised me to leave Kampen. A few weeks later Kampen became the place
where the German occupation authorities landed 8000 men picked up in round-
ups in Rotterdam; they had been transported by boat across the IJsselmeer to
be transported to Germany. This event challenged Kolff to employ all his
diplomatic skills to do something for these round-up victims, as will be
described in Chapter 7. New responsibilities demanded all his time and attention. All work on the artificial kidney came to a standstill until the end of
World War II in Europe.

4.1 ALL THE THINGS WE DID NOT HAVE

'Antibiotics' was a notion nobody knew in the Netherlands in 1943–44. Sulphonamides were the only drugs active against some species of bacteria. They only inhibited the growth of bacteria that do not form pus; hence they had no effect on, *inter alia*, staphylococci. Some sulphonamides, e.g. sulphapyridine, became notorious because they tended to crystallize in the renal passages and hence block the flow of urine. That was actually the case with patient number 10, the first one to recover completely after a dialysis.

Patient number 7 would probably never have been treated with the artificial kidney if penicillin had been available. he developed a staphylococcal abscess in his right kidney and it was removed surgically. Uraemia developed and he was brought to Kampen where he was dialysed twice. He ran a high fever during the second dialysis: he was delirious and tried to pull the needles out of his arms. He died the morning after the dialysis. At autopsy he was found to be one of those very rare persons who are born without a functioning left kidney!

Soap became scarcer and scarcer. The modern detergents which are so common nowadays did not yet exist. Another group of materials which were non-existent was the whole group of plastics which are so common nowadays. Rubber tubing, glass tubing and tape were the materials we had to depend on – all from a stock that could not be replenished. No disposable tubing or needles were available for blood transfusions: the technician of the Central Laboratory of the Red Cross in Amsterdam taught me carefully how a needle used for a transfusion could be made suitable for a subsequent transfusion after removing all traces of blood.

Determination of the potassium level of the blood plasma of patients likely to be treated with dialysis was very important: both an abnormally high and an abnormally low potassium level could have very serious consequences for the heart. Unfortunately the method for determining potassium that was available then was very time-consuming; it was very sensitive to disturbing factors. Much later the flame photometer, developed after World War II, made determination of potassium a matter of a few minutes!

Can you imagine a hospital without a single computer? Such a one was the hospital where the artificial kidney was developed. The text of all Kolff's publications was composed at night in Kolff's home – without a textwriter program! I was lucky enough to possess a simple portable typewriter and that served us admirably in writing the first papers on the artificial kidney. It was a great advantage that Kolff did not have to do the typing himself: the person typing a text himself is somewhat more reticent in making changes than the person who leaves the typing to someone else. The reason is that not a single word could be crossed out or inserted or moved to another place in the sentence without leaving a trace (I had no correction fluid at my disposal). Typing without errors was a skill that was held in very high esteem at that time – any change in the text meant that the page had to be typed again before a neat final version was reached. A textwriter program that makes it possible to develop a text from 'thinking aloud' to a crystal-clear story was something nobody could dream of at that time!

Something one never heard was the request 'Just make a copy, will you?' Photocopy machines like the ones we are familiar with did not exist. Kolff had bought a photocopying machine himself and had it installed in the darkroom of the x-ray room of the hospital. It used light-sensitive paper that had to be exposed, developed, fixed, washed and dried to provide a negative. When dry this was used to make a positive image on a second sheet of paper. Washing lines along the wall of the dark room were used to dry the sheets. Persons entering the darkroom when we were busy were often shocked at so many rows of sheets of paper, like death announcements, hanging there: the original documents were usually smaller than the photographic paper, so that the copies had solemn black borders. It was a time when the newspapers could at any time have an obituary on the front page concerning one or more persons shot by the German occupation forces for deeds of resistance or just as a hostage – events which the generations born after World War II may have heard of, but which fortunately do not arouse the emotions which we felt at that time.

5

THE FIRST SERIES OF 17 PATIENTS

When the first artificial kidney was completed at the end of 1942 it was clear that the medical practitioners in and around Kampen would have to acquire sufficient confidence in this new development to refer kidney patients to Kolff – unless the kidney by chance became a reasonable option for a patient who had already been admitted to the Kampen hospital. It would not be easy to develop such a confidence without any experience with the treatment of patients. In fact it was a kind of chicken-and-egg problem.

Fortunately Kolff had established good relationships with the general practitioners in the Kampen area and with the specialists in Zwolle, the nearest larger town. In December 1942 the ophthalmologist Dr Keiner in Zwolle was visited by a young woman with progressively deteriorating sight. The cause proved to be a chronic nephritis with hypertension. She was referred to Kolff via the internist Dhont in Zwolle for treatment with the kidney. She was in a bad condition at that time; she vomited repeatedly. Dhont knew that there was nothing to lose, but perhaps a temporary improvement could be attained.

In fact Kolff had had another type of patient in mind when he tackled the development of an artificial kidney. He had thought in the first place of patients with temporary kidney trouble who might be helped to overcome a critical period, after which their own kidneys would resume their task again. The hope of achieving a temporary improvement was the argument in this case to start the lady's treatment.

Her history has been described *in extenso* in Kolff's doctoral thesis.[1] She was connected to the artificial kidney 12 times from 17 March onwards: the first time this lasted only 22 minutes. When this showed that she could tolerate this treatment well the dialyses became longer and longer: the tenth one lasted 6 hours. From the seventh to the tenth dialysis her condition improved so much directly after the dialysis that she vomited less and became clearer in her mind.

All types of complications occurred. Some lots of the heparin that was used to keep the blood from clotting outside her body caused febrile reactions. The removal of the needle from the artery after the seventh dialysis caused a very persistent haemorrhage. That was the time when Kolff showed his leadership by facing all the complications with a sober mind, learning from setbacks and devising another strategy for the next time. Kolff used the experiences with this patient in three different ways.

He used them in the first paper on the artificial kidney 'De Kunstmatige Nier, een Dialysator met groot oppervlak' ('The artificial kidney, a dialyser with a great area'), which appeared on 27 August 1943; the authors were W. J. Kolff and H. Th. J. Berk, and the assistance was acknowledged of Sister M. ter Welle, Miss A. J. W. van der Leij (the technician who did all the determinations), E. C. van Dijk (the engineer from the Kampen Enamel Works) and J. van Noordwijk.[2] Secondly, Kolff used the experience to build a second, larger, kidney which will be dealt with more fully in the following chapter. Thirdly, he used this experience to make this new type of treatment better known at clinical meetings.

In this way he could build up experience with the treatment of another 14 patients between May 1943 and the end of August 1944: three of them were treated in the Municipal Hospital of The Hague and two in Amsterdam (they are also described in the following chapter). Thirteen of these died soon after treatment with the kidney. As to the only patient who recovered completely Kolff declared that he also had a good chance of recovery without this treatment. How can it be explained then that Kolff built up so much confidence that his colleagues continued to refer patients to him?

A positive factor was that Kolff did not present the results of these treatments as more favourable than they in fact were. In addition, the failure of the patients' own kidneys was in many cases due to a pathological process for which no efficient treatment was known. Two patients had cancer of the kidneys or the bladder, one had tuberculosis of the kidneys and the bladder – we lived in an era in which no antibiotics or chemotherapy against tuberculosis was known. Two patients died as a result of intoxication with bichloride of mercury: it was only after the liberation that dimercaprol became available as a specific antidote against mercury intoxication. Patients with acute nephritis often developed a pneumonia which could be only poorly treated with the chemotherapy known at that time (only sulfa drugs).

On the other hand the condition of a number of patients clearly improved during or soon after the renal dialysis, even if this was only a temporary improvement. In addition Kolff could demonstrate how the technique improved on the basis of experience.

The way in which the method of connecting the kidney to the patient's blood vessels was improved step by step has already been described.

A second problem was the dose of heparin needed to keep the blood from clotting as long as it circulated through the kidney. When too little heparin was used clotting occurred; when too much heparin was used the vessels used to make the connection continued to bleed afterwards. In this respect, too, the transition to glass cannulae was an improvement: the risk of clotting decreased, and sometimes they could remain *in situ* so that they could also be used for intravenous infusions after the dialysis.

A third problem was mechanical damage of the erythrocytes (haemolysis). This gave no problems in the first patient: it became a problem only when the kidney was assembled some time before dialysis, and the cellophane tube was kept from drying out and shrinking, with glycerine. We solved the problem by adding glucose to the dialysing fluid to a concentration of 1.5% and by limiting the use of glycerine (as described in the preceding chapter).

Starting with the second patient a dialysis always lasted at least 6 hours. The amount of urea demonstrable in the bath then corresponded with 1.5–8 times the 24-hour excretion of a normal adult. The long duration of these treatments also increased the chance, of course, that not only the urea concentration but also that of other constituents of the blood plasma would change. Sometimes Kolff used this in a positive way: he succeeded, for example, in withdrawing fluid from the body in the case of patient 7 by raising the glucose concentration of the dialysing fluid, thus diminishing his oedema. In other cases it became apparent after the dialysis that there had been insufficient control of the sodium and potassium ion concentration, although these are vital for the salt and water balance of the body. As mentioned before, this was partly due to the fact that the determination of the sodium and potassium content of the blood took a long time in those years; in addition the presence of heparin often interfered with the determination of potassium. However, heparin was indispensable, to keep the blood from clotting.

Due to the sensible optimism of Kolff and the devotion of his co-workers it was possible to treat 15 patients with the kidney in about a year and a half.

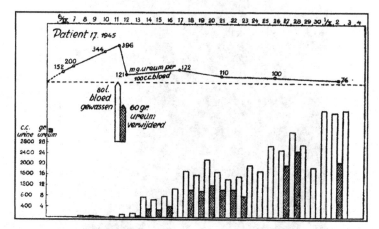

Figure 5.1 The clinical chemical picture of patient 17, the first one who owed her life to the artificial kidney. The graph at the top represents the urea content of her blood before and after the dialysis. The vertical arrow indicates the 80 litres of blood that flowed through the artificial kidney, the shaded arrow the 60 grams of urea that were removed.

The open rectangles indicate the volume of urine passed by the patient, the shaded ones the grams of urea she excreted. (From the MD thesis of W. J. Kolff.)

The experience gained in this way contributed markedly in 1945 to the successful treatment of a woman suffering from both a cholecystitis with a pericholecys-
titis and a nephritis.

She was in a coma when she was connected to the kidney. She awoke during
the dialysis and began to talk of what she planned to do in the future: obtain
a divorce from her husband – which in fact she did when she had recovered.
Figure 5.1 shows her blood urea level before and after the dialysis, and also
the recovery of her own renal function. Shortly after the dialysis she was up
and about again (see Figure 5.2).

Her plans for the future had another special aspect: she had been interned
after the end of the war as a political offender, and she had been taken to

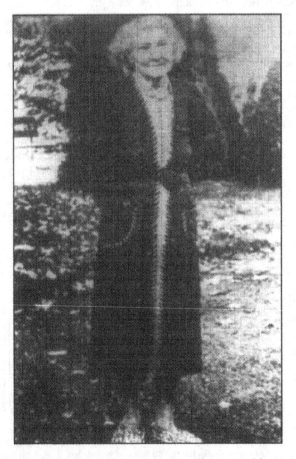

Figure 5.2   Mrs Sophie Schafstadt, the first patient whose life was saved by treatment with the
artificial kidney. Her dialysis started on 11 September 1945 and continued for 11.5 hours.

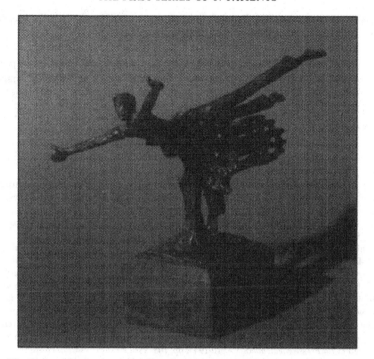

Figure 5.3 The patient floating towards a new future after treatment with the artificial kidney, seen through the eyes of the American sculptor Dennis Smith.

hospital from the military barracks in Kampen where political offenders were kept prisoner at that time.[3] The commander-in-chief of those barracks, Mr Oudshoorn, proved to be an old acquaintance of Kolff: during the German occupation Oudshoorn had been active in the underground resistance movement, and Kolff had seen to it then that he had symptoms of a disease which kept him from being sent to work in Germany by the occupation forces.

Oudshoorn was willing to let this lady stay in hospital and then let her go to one of her sons (one of her sons had also been active in the underground resistance during the occupation, another son had been interned after the war because of collaboration with the Nazis). She made a complete recovery there. Six years later she died from another disease at the age of 73.

When it became clear, in September 1945, that she was going to recover, the first half of Kolff's doctorate thesis had already been typeset: fortunately he was able to include her treatment under 'Conclusion' just before the 'Summary':

The 67-year-old woman just described made such a serious impression before the dialysis that her death was imminent. I am convinced that she would have died if the treatment with the artificial kidney had not taken place. If others agree with me this would have made it likely that it is possible to save the life of some patients suffering from acute uraemia with the help of vividialysis. An incitement to continue along this route.

The leap towards a new future which dialysis may make possible has been expressed by the American sculptor Dennis Smith in the small statuette which he made at Kolff's request many decades later. To express his gratitude Kolff gave copies to his co-workers who had supported him in these first years, in his efforts to show that dialysis may open a new future for kidney patients (see Figure 5.3).

NOTES

1. Kolff WJ. De kunstmatige nier (The artificial kidney). Thesis for obtaining the doctorate in medicine at the University of Groningen, 16 January 1946. Promoter was Professor R. Brinkman, MD.
2. Kolff WJ, Berk HThJ, with the cooperation of Sister M. ter Welle, Miss A. J. W. van der Leij, E. C. van Dijk and J. van Noordwijk. The artificial kidney: a dialyser with a great area (In Dutch). *Geneeskundige Gids* 1943; 21 (number 21), 27 August. An abbreviated version was published under the same title and with the same authors and co-workers in the *Nederlands Tijdschrift voor Geneeskunde* in 1943; 87: 1684–1687. The same authors published an article in English under the title 'The artificial kidney: a dialyser with a great area' in the Swedish journal *Acta Medica Scandinavica*, 1944; 117: 121–134. This contained a postscript dated 15 January 1944 with a summary of the results obtained with the second and third patients. The importance of this publication was mainly that it was also distributed in those countries that were not occupied by Germany, Italy or Japan. Finally a brief article by the same authors in French appeared in *La Presse Médicale* of 8 April 1944, pp. 103–110.
3. Thorwald J. *Die Patienten: Die Helden dieses Buches sind Menschen wie Du und ich.* Droemer: Knauer, 1970.

THE SECOND AND THIRD ARTIFICIAL KIDNEY

6.1 TECHNICAL DEVELOPMENTS IN THE APPARATUS

When the rotating artificial kidney basically proved to function well Kolff decided to have a second, larger, apparatus built. That was not so simple: the Kampen Enamel Works were no longer able to furnish anything more than the enamel tank. Fortunately Kolff was able to secure the cooperation of several other persons.

Aluminium plate, the material from which the drum of the kidney had been made, was no longer obtainable. A local cartwright built an open cylinder of beech wood slats of about 1 cm thick and about 1 cm of space between them. The rotation of such a drum no longer caused a soft rustling such as the first kidney did, but a clear splashing. This was muffled when a leak arose in the cellophane tube allowing blood to enter the dialysing fluid, causing clouds of foam to overflow the rim of the tank on to the floor.

The chassis of the second kidney was also built of wood (see Figure 6.1). It had a height of 80 cm and hence the apparatus was easier to handle with the continuous perfusion which had come into use in the meantime.

Mr Harmsen, the head of the Laboratory of the Northeast Polder (the polder reclaimed from the eastern part of the IJsselmeer) contributed by having his glassblower make glass cannulae and other glassware. Kolff also sought the help of Mr J. Snoep, the director of the engineering works 'De IJssel', and invited him to see the artificial kidney in action. Mr Snoep recorded his impressions in a rather original way (see Figure 6.2), but he also assisted with several metal constructions, which the Kampen Enamel Works could no longer supply because of the closer and closer German supervision. To our regret Mr Snoep could not witness the development of the artificial kidney after the war. He was arrested by the Germans because he was suspected of underground resistance activities, and he was shot shortly after.

The continuous perfusion from an artery made it necessary to speed up the return of the blood to the patient; this made it necessary to obtain a pump. Several small tube pumps for manual operation were on the market for blood transfusion; small rollers compressing a rubber tube moved on the blood inside the tube. However, they were intended only for short-time use. When I rotated such a tube by hand for an hour the rubber tube was worn away, and that

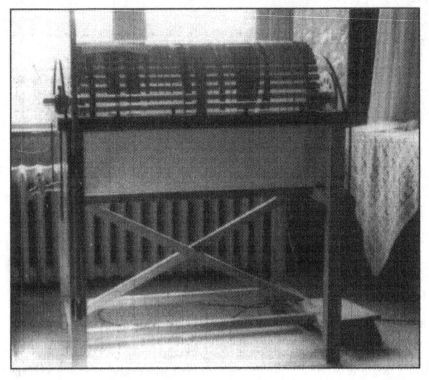

Figure 6.1   The second artificial kidney: the cylinder and the frame were made out of wood by a local cartwright. The Kamper Email Fabrieken (Kampen Enamel Works) again made the enamel tank.

made it clear that these pumps were not suitable for our purpose. The original tube pump, designed by Beck, had rollers with a much larger diameter, and they proved to damage the rubber tube far less, if at all. Hence a pump of similar design was used in the second and following kidneys and driven from the axle of the rotating drum.

Leaks in the cellophane tube could cause air bubbles to enter the patient's circulation, and to prevent this we introduced a bubble trap: a vertical glass tube, closed at the lower end by a rubber stopper with two short tubes for the inflow and outflow of the blood. Any air bubbles would be trapped in the upper end of the tube.

The third artificial kidney was similar to the second one, except that the chassis was no longer built of wood: it was a metal framework on castors.

6.2   THE FIRST KIDNEY GOES TO THE HAGUE

The construction of the second kidney not only gave us an apparatus with a greater power, but it also provided the opportunity to install the first one in

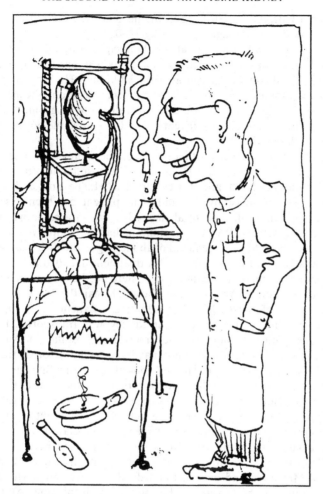

Figure 6.2 Kolff and the artificial kidney: an impression by Mr J. Snoep.

The Hague. Transportation of patients to Kampen for treatment with the kidney was difficult at that time; therefore Kolff aimed at making such treatment available elsewhere.

The need for that became apparent after the monthly magazine *Geneeskundige Gids* (the Medical Guide) had published the first paper on the treatment of the first patient. A paper on this subject appeared in the *Nederlands Tijdschrift voor Geneeskunde* (the Netherlands Medical Journal) in November 1943, and this led to new requests in the following months to treat patients with this apparatus.

When the second kidney was operational in Kampen the first one went to the Municipal Hospital in The Hague, the hospital where Kolff had installed the blood bank during the fighting in May 1940.

In the summer of 1943 I arrived at this Municipal Hospital with the kidney in a small delivery van. I informed the porter, as if it was the most common message, that I had come to deliver an artificial kidney. His reaction surprised me: 'For which firm are you coming to give a demonstration?', he asked. I was indignant: just imagine, I had not come to sell something, but to help the hospital to an important medical invention! But of course the porter could not be expected to know this.

In November 1943 a patient with an acute glomerulonephritis was admitted to the medical department of Dr Holmer in that hospital, for treatment with the artificial kidney. Kolff and I went to The Hague and a dialysis was performed, closely watched by the staff. This patient has been described as patient number 3 in Kolff's doctoral thesis. He was in a coma when he was connected to the kidney. When his condition had not improved after more than 7½ hours – in spite of the removal of about 80 g of urea – it was concluded that there was no point in prolonging this treatment. He died a day later.

This kidney also made a journey to Amsterdam, before the third kidney could be installed there. An emergency hospital near the Vondel Park (just outside the centre of Amsterdam) had admitted a patient for whom dialysis appeared to be indicated. Therefore the kidney was transported from The Hague to the patient's room in the emergency hospital in Amsterdam. Unfortunately this institution did not have the facilities for sterilizing the components of the blood circuit. Hence I took them to the 'Binnengasthuis' (a hospital in the centre of Amsterdam), to the attic where the Central Laboratory of the Red Cross Blood Transfusion had been installed. All rubber tubes, glass connecting pieces and the cellophane tube were cleaned and put in a large pan; this was wrapped up in strong packing paper and autoclaved.

With that parcel under my arm I took the tram to the emergency hospital near the Vondel Park. The atmosphere was tense in Amsterdam at that time: the strike of May 1943 had only just ended,[1] the air was alive with rumours of new round-ups by the Germans – but all went well this time. All the same I preferred to stay on the rear open balcony of the tram with the kidney underneath my arm, so that I would be able to get off quickly if necessary. Assembling the kidney caused no problems.

Eventually all this need not have been done, for the patient's kidney function recovered so that dialysis was not necessary.

6.3 THE THIRD KIDNEY GOES TO AMSTERDAM

The third kidney was completed in the autumn of 1943. It was wheeled on to the night boat and I accompanied it from Kampen to Amsterdam, to bring it to the Central Laboratory of the Red Cross Blood Transfusion Service under the care of Dr J. Spaander.[2]

Patients number 4 and 6, described by Kolff in his doctoral thesis, were treated in Amsterdam. Patient number 6, a woman with acute glomerulonephritis as a complication of scarlet fever, was treated in an emergency hospital in the southern part of Amsterdam. The transportation of the kidney from Dr Spaander's laboratory to that hospital caused no problems, but when the patient had to be wheeled into the room where the kidney was set up her bed could not pass through the door opening. A carpenter had to be fetched first to break away part of the doorpost before she could be connected to the kidney. (In those days my doctor's bag did contain electrician's pliers and a set of screwdrivers, but no crowbar.)

The patient's condition improved during the dialysis: her drowsiness decreased, and she started to tell of her family. Two days after the dialysis her own diuresis started to return, but unfortunately she died a day later from a pneumonia.

NOTES

1. General Christiansen, the German commander in the Netherlands, announced on Thursday 29 April 1943 that all Dutch military personnel had to report as prisoners of war. The reaction was the outbreak of a spontaneous strike in the largest factory of Hengelo, the engineering works of the Stork Brothers, on the same day. The next day strikes started all over the Netherlands. The SS general Rauter reacted by proclaiming police summary justice for several regions. That implied that sentences of death could be proclaimed and executed as under martial law. A total of 116 sentences of death were pronounced in the following days: 80 executions were carried out. In Marum, in the province of Groningen, 16 people were arrested and shot without any further hearing. For more details consult the book by L. de Jong *The History of the Kingdom of the Netherlands in the Second World War* (in Dutch), volume 6, second half. Of course the situation also remained turbulent after the state of police summary justice had ended on 15 May.
2. Kolff and Spaander had kept up contact as a result of Kolff's organization of a blood bank in The Hague during the May days of 1940. The possibility to clean and sterilize materials for the artificial kidney in the Central Laboratory of the Blood Transfusion Service in Amsterdam was very welcome when Kolff wanted to make treatment with the kidney possible in more locations in the Netherlands.

7
HIBERNATION OF THE KIDNEY 1944–1945

When it became clear that the second kidney essentially met all Kolff's expectations he had a series of four kidneys built, of the same type as the third kidney; that is kidneys with a metal frame and casters. They were finished at the beginning of 1944, and their photograph decorates the beginning of Kolff's doctoral thesis (see Figure 7.1).

The landing of the allied troops in Normandy in June 1944 not only raised hopes in all of us that we would soon be liberated, but it also caused Kolff to worry that these four kidneys might become lost as a result of local armed actions at the liberation. Therefore he took care to store them in different places, so as to increase the chance that at least a few of them would survive the war.

After the fifteenth patient had been treated the approach of the war front put an end to the application of the artificial kidney in Kampen. The rumours inspired Mr Schilder, one of the patients in the men's ward, to sketch his idea of the hospital staff taking part in the triumphal procession after the liberation from the German occupation: it is shown in Figure 7.2. In September 1944 rumours began to spread that the allied troops were advancing rapidly, culminating in rumours that the allies would be in the Netherlands within a few hours on Tuesday 5 September, the day that has become known in this country as 'Dolle Dinsdag' (Crazy Tuesday). When these rumours proved to be false the German army started to speed up the building of defence works, and held round-ups to compel Dutchmen to work on them.

On the morning of Saturday 16 September Kolff said to me 'Bob, I expect trouble here. You'd better disappear. Go to my father's sanatorium in Beekbergen.' Beekbergen is situated just north of Arnhem. A sanatorium was a relatively safe place, for German troops were so scared of tuberculosis that they kept away from any places where tuberculosis was bound to be present.

I went to my room, packed a few clothes and left on my bicycle. On the way I was warned that the Germans were holding a round-up near Apeldoorn, but I could take a side road and I arrived safely in Beekbergen.

The next morning, Sunday 17 September, we heard gunfire: allied airborne troops had landed at Oosterbeek just west of Arnhem as part of the operation 'Market Garden'. The result of that operation is well known now. A few days

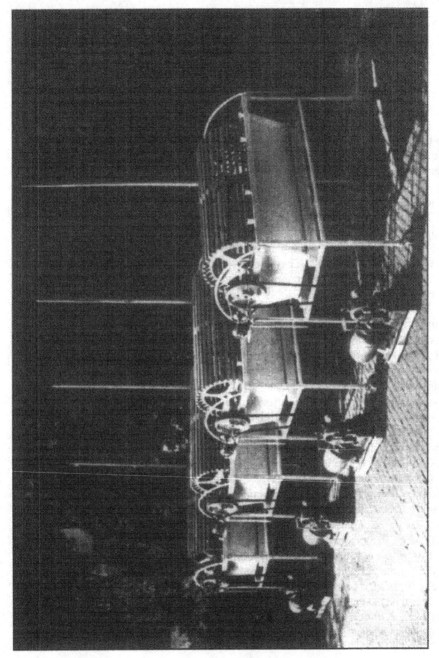

Figure 7.1   The first series of four artificial kidneys delivered in September 1944. (From the MD thesis of W. J. Kolff.)

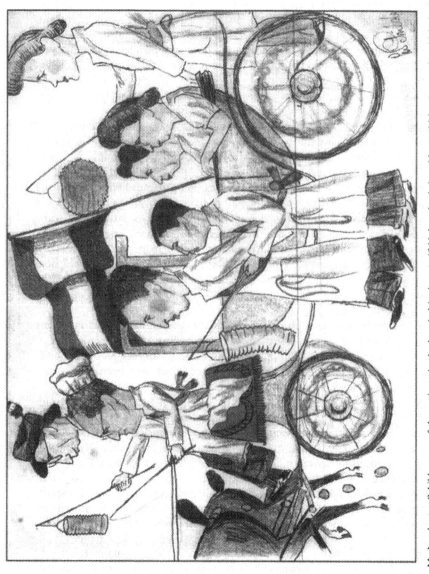

Figure 7.2 Mr Lambertus Schilder, one of the patients in the hospital in August 1944, imagined that this would be the way in which the hospital staff would take part in the procession to celebrate the liberation from the German occupation. Sitting on the coach-box Dr Kolff and the director Dr J. K. W. Kehrer; in the carriage Sister Ter Welle and Sister Koezen, behind them in attendance Miss Nannie K. M. de Leeuw; the senior medical student L. de Jong and the internist Dr K. B. Tjook, who worked in the department of internal medicine in 1944, walk alongside.

later it became clear to us that our liberation would not come within a few days, and I decided to leave the Kolff family in Beekbergen. I wanted to go to Groningen to await the end of the war there at the home of my future parents-in-law, Mr and Mrs Van Veen.

Near Apeldoorn I was warned again that the Germans were holding a round-up. This time a farmer let me hide in his haystack. The next morning the coast was clear again, and I cycled to Kampen without any problem. The situation there was such that it would be unsafe for me to stay. The Germans controlled the bridge across the IJssel river and checked everyone's papers, except on Thursday, because that was market day in Kampen. Luckily it was Thursday, and I reached the other side of the river without being stopped.

Without meeting any Germans I reached Blankenham where I stayed over-night with relatives of my future father-in-law and continued my trip next day. All went well until I reached Leek, some 10 km west of Groningen: I was stopped by three members of the 'Landwacht', the Dutch national-socialist rural police. When they asked me where I was going I told them I was on my way to Professor Brinkman with information from the firm of Organon. I did in fact have official papers as an employee of that firm because I did some biochemical research for Professor Brinkman; as Organon did work for the German army that had protected me from being called up for work in Germany.

The 'Landwacht' let me go. Only a quarter of an hour later I realized how lucky I was that they had been as little conscious as I had been about the advance of the allies: the firm of Organon in Oss had been liberated by allied troops a few days before!

I reached the home of my future parents-in-law in Groningen about a quarter of an hour before curfew time and remained in hiding there until the end of the war (16 April 1945 for Groningen). This made it possible for me to back out of the obligation to dig trenches for defence which had been proclaimed by the German commander for all men in Groningen.

In November the Germans held large round-ups in Rotterdam to pick up men for work in Germany. Because allied planes bombarded the railway lines the Germans transported their victims in flat-bottom ships across the IJsselmeer from Amsterdam to Kampen, and on 11 November more than 10 000 victims of these round-ups were made to debark in Kampen. Soon after Dr Pel, one of the general practitioners who lived on the quayside, phoned Kolff that horrible things had taken place. The German commander of this transport, Oberleutnant Ernst Baatz, personally shot one of the victims, the Jewish citizen Abraham van der Schoot who had been in hiding when the round-up took place; his body was thrown in the river. Pel urged Kolff to do something.

Kolff went up to Baatz: 'he was drunk, but he was not unfair', Kolff said later.[1] Kolff managed to persuade him that prisoners that were seriously ill could not work for Baatz anyway, and asked permission to take out the most seriously ill men and convey them to the town hospital and emergency hospitals. Baatz demanded that Kolff first get permission from Mr E. F. Sandberg, the national socialist burgomaster of Kampen, appointed by the Germans in 1942. Kolff refused, saying he had nothing to do with Sandberg. 'You will be shot if anyone escapes, Mr Kolff!' was the reply of Baatz – but he let Kolff select 800 seriously ill.

They were transported to the town hospital and to emergency hospitals all led by a local doctor. Dr Kehrer, the director of the town hospital, was responsible. He and Kolff kept an accurate administration. Among them were members of resistance groups that had been trapped by the round-up in Rotterdam: they falsified ration cards and personal papers, and theoretically the administration was perfect. When they started to falsify their own personal papers in order to escape Kolff persuaded them that no-one should leave the hospital or any of the emergency hospitals on his own, because that would endanger the persons staying behind.

However, the most serious danger for Kolff did not come from the side of the German officials, but from Sandberg. Ever since he came to Kampen in 1942 he had been ignored by the hospital. Sandberg urged Baatz every day to make surprise visits to the hospital because hospitals were the centres of all kinds of illegal activities. Kolff heard of this, and to be ahead of him Kehrer and Kolff invited Baatz and his staff for an official visit. Kolff showed the artificial kidney to the senior medical officer, who said 'Yes, that is the apparatus I already know from the literature'.[2] Whether that was true or not will always remain a mystery: it could be true, for the Swedish journal *Acta Medica Scandinavica* carried an article on the kidney in the spring of 1944. In any case it helped to lessen the suspicion of the German authorities.

When the visitors entered a ward full of epileptics one of them developed an attack. Other patients followed, and this whole ward full of tonic and clonic convulsing bodies convinced Baatz, at least for the time being, that the persons in that ward really were patients. Baatz told Kolff later that Sandberg had tried to convince him again that Kolff tried to cheat him; when Kolff asked Baatz what his reply had been, Baatz said 'I only grinned in his face.'

Working with the artificial kidney had to be postponed until after the liberation. For Kampen that took place on 17 April 1945.

NOTES

1. Kolff told this in the NOS television programme broadcast in February 1989 as part of the programme series 'Markant'.
2. Weisse AB. Turning bad luck into good: the alchemy of Willem Johan Kolff. *Seminars in Dialysis*, 1993; 6: 52–58. Weisse also relates how Snapper landed in New York. He left Amsterdam in 1938 so as not to come under a national socialist regime: he had been appointed as professor of internal medicine in 1919 when he was 30 years old! He landed in China at the Peiping Union Medical College. There he fell into the hands of the Japanese, but he was exchanged against a Japanese general who had fallen into the hands of the Dutch. He arrived in the United States where he was employed at the Mount Sinai Hospital in New York from 1944 to 1952.

8

RECOGNITION AT HOME AND ABROAD

'This thesis describes a study aimed at a well defined goal: the construction of an artificial kidney and the adaptation of this apparatus to its use in the clinic.' That is the opening sentence of the introduction to the doctoral thesis[1] which Kolff defended to obtain the degree of doctor of medicine at the University of Groningen on 16 January 1946. Professor R. Brinkman was his promoter.

The author of a thesis traditionally uses the introduction to express his gratitude to the persons who have rendered important contributions to the study described in the thesis. Kolff did so too, and mentioned in the first place Mr H. Th. J. Berk and Mr E. C. van Dijk, the director and the draughtsman and engineer of the Kamper Email Fabrieken (Kampen Enamel Works); and then Mr E. W. F. Hammers as one of those who helped to construct new kidneys when that had become impossible in the Kamper Email Fabrieken due to tighter supervision by the occupation authorities. Attention is then drawn by the sentence: 'Outside of the town of Kampen I have also received much support, from my brother C. Kolff, from several Governmental Bureaux, from manufacturers and laboratories when the objective was to obtain or produce machines or components for the kidney to the detriment of supplies to the German Wehrmacht.'

Quite rightly Kolff thanked the nurses: 'My head nurse Sister M. ter Welle has been a great support in this work, for the artificial kidney has placed a heavy extra burden on the shoulders of the nurses of the Municipal Hospital of Kampen. I can say that they all have helped enthusiastically; they have kept watch many nights and did not count their fatigue.' The two chemical technicians, Miss A. J. W. van der Leij and Miss W. Eskes, are also thanked: 'they have carried out almost all the determinations mentioned in this thesis and hundreds of others that were directed more or less towards working with the kidney' (see Figure 8.1). They had always been willing to do chemical analyses whatever the time of day or night.

The first of the theses added to the manuscript may be read as a triumphant conclusion of the whole study: 'Acute uraemia may now be combated successfully; it need no longer be the primary cause of death of a patient.'

A spirited three-quarters of an hour of attack and defence of the doctoral thesis and the theses was followed by the decision of the Senate to award to

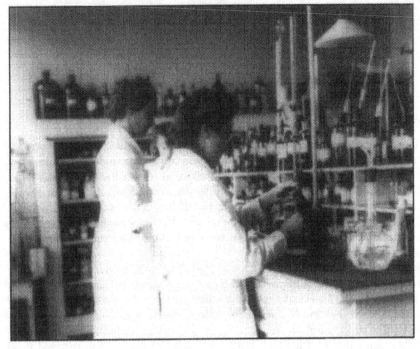

Figure 8.1   Miss A. J. W. ('Mieneke') van der Leij and Miss W. ('Willy') Eskes in the laboratory where all the chemical determinations for the dialyses in Kampen were carried out.

him the doctorate in medicine with the qualification 'cum laude', to the great joy of all the co-workers from Kampen who were able to attend this extraordinary event.

Here too Kolff showed his ability to break with obsolete traditions. Traditionally the 'young doctor' (as he was called on that occasion) offers a dinner to which only his male study friends are invited – 1½ years later I was still invited to such an event in Groningen. Kolff broke with this tradition: instead he organized a buffet in a restaurant where Sister M. ter Welle and all the other co-workers from Kampen were cordially welcome: a festive award for their contributions to the development of the artificial kidney (see Figure 8.2). The whole staff of the hospital could not attend the reception, of course, but they soon found an occasion to celebrate the end of the war and the beginning of a new era in medicine (see Figure 8.3).

This doctoral thesis, of course, further publicized Kolff's work in the Netherlands – but what about making it known abroad? In the sixteenth century Erasmus only needed to write *In praise of folly* in Latin to make it known all over Europe. Before World War II the German language served as 'the language of science' in many ways, but English was slowly becoming more

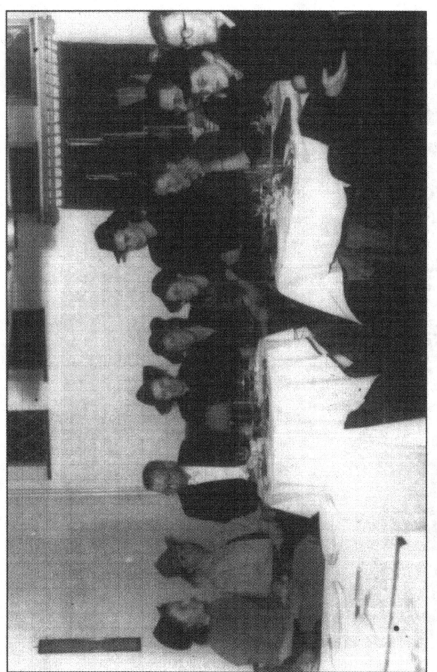

Figure 8.2 The whole 'kidney team' from Kampen visited the reception after Kolff had obtained his MD on 16 January 1946. From left to right: Miss A. (Ant) Vlaanderen, secretary; Sister M. ter Welle, Nurse J. Raab and Nurse G. van den Noort, Miss W. (Willy) Eskes and Miss A. J. W. (Mieneke) van der Leij, Miss N. K. M. (Nannie) de Leeuw (resident), Mr L. van Dellén (the fiancé of Miss Van der Leij) and the author with his fiancée Miss J. C. van Veen.

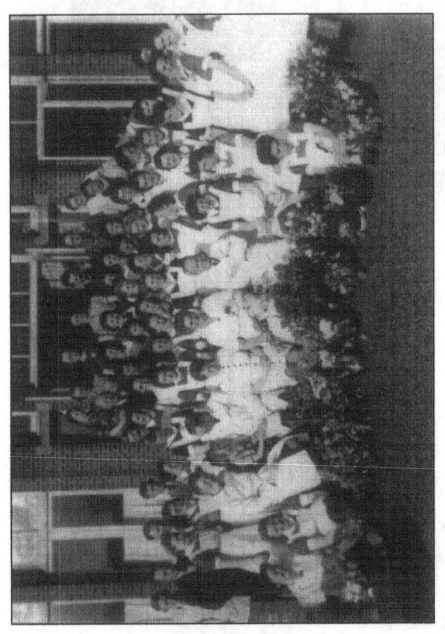

Figure 8.3 The staff of the hospital in the spring of 1946. Sitting on the first row the Director Dr J. K. W. Kehrer, to his left sister Koeczen, Ms I. van der Wal (head of the housekeeping department); next to her Dr W. J. Kolff with his daughter Adrie and Ms N. K. M. (Nannie) de Leeuw. To the right of Dr Kehrer are Nurses J. Raab and G. van den Noort.

and more the language of leading journals. Medical researchers in Scandinavia set up *Acta Medica Scandinavica*, a journal that published papers in English; thus they could be read much more widely than if they had been published in Swedish, Danish, Norwegian, Finnish or Icelandic. We were told that hospital interns in England read articles in this journal aloud to each other over breakfast to make fun of the funny English of those foreigners. Kolff did not mind that: 'Then they read these articles at least', was his comment.

An additional advantage of *Acta Medica Scandinavica* during World War II was that it was obtainable both in the Netherlands and in the free world not occupied by the Germans. That is why Kolff had offered his first publication on the artificial kidney in English to this journal in 1943. It appeared at the beginning of 1944 under the title: 'The artificial kidney: a dialyser with a great area'.[2]

Directly after the liberation of the Netherlands in 1945 I had resumed my study of medicine in Groningen, but at the request of Kolff I assisted in making a shortened version of his doctoral thesis in English. He entrusted me with this task because I had had the good luck to go to school in London for two years, in the period when my father was stationed there from 1929 until 1932. This English version was published in 1946 under the title *The Artificial Kidney*, by Dr W. J. Kolff with the cooperation of J. van Noordwijk[3] (see Figure 8.4). Kolff sent copies to all the authors he could reach whose work he had cited in his doctoral thesis.

Immediately after the end of the war Kolff asked the British Information Service in The Hague whether they had any information on developments in the free world concerning dialysis, but this service had nothing to report. In fact the first paper by Alwall in Sweden on his artificial kidney only appeared in 1947;[4] Gordon Murray in Toronto published his results with an artificial kidney only in 1948[5] (see Figure 8.5).

Kolff collected his four kidneys from their hiding places and sent them out into the world. One he gave to the Hammersmith Hospital in London under the care of Dr Bywaters and Dr Joekes. A second one he gave to a hospital in Poland; he lost sight of it, but news came in 1977 that it had turned up in Cracow.[6] The third kidney he gave to the Mount Sinai Hospital in New York, under the care of Professor Snapper. The fourth one was donated to the Royal Victoria Hospital in Montreal, and what happened with it is described in Chapter 10.

Professor Snapper invited Kolff for a series of lectures in the United States.[7]

This interest abroad led to new copies of the second version of the kidney on the basis of technical drawings of it in Kolff's doctoral thesis. This took place in London (Ontario) in Canada, and in Boston and Milwaukee in the United States. In the meantime other ways of treating kidney patients were being developed in the Netherlands.

THE ARTIFICIAL KIDNEY

BY

Dr W. J. KOLFF

INTERNIST OF THE MUNICIPAL HOSPITAL "ENGELENBERGSTICHTING"
KAMPEN (HOLLAND)

WITH THE COOPERATION OF
J. VAN NOORDWIJK
Med. Drs

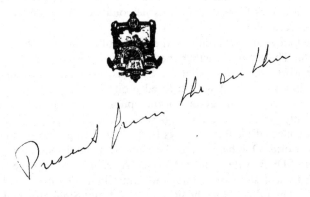

J. H. KOK N.V. KAMPEN (HOLLAND) 1946

Figure 8.4 The title page of the English abbreviated version of W. J. Kolff's MD thesis: he sent copies of this to all authors abroad whom he had cited in his text.

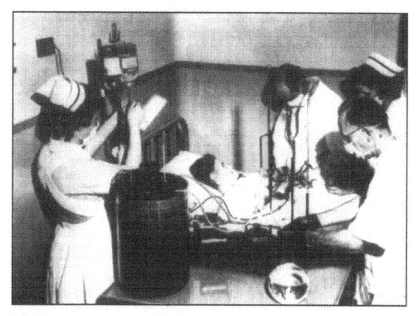

Figure 8.5 Dr Gordon Murray (on the right) adjusting the pump of the artificial kidney he had developed in Toronto.

NOTES

1. Kolff WJ. De kunstmatige nier (The artificial kidney). Thesis for obtaining the doctorate in medicine at the University of Groningen, 16 January 1946. Promoter was Professor R. Brinkman.
2. Kolff WJ, Berk H Th J, with the collaboration of Nurse M. ter Welle, Miss A. J. W. van der Leij, E. C. van Dijk and J. van Noordwijk. The artificial kidney: a dialyser with a great area. *Acta Medica Scandinavica*, 1944; 117: 121–134.
3. Kolff WJ with the cooperation of J. van Noordwijk. *The Artificial Kidney*. Kampen: J. H. Kok NV, 1946.
4. Alwall N. On the artificial Kidney. I. Apparatus for dialysis of blood *in vivo*. *Acta Medica Scandinavica* 1947; 128: 317. See also Alwall N, Norviit L. On the artificial kidney II. The effectivity of the apparatus. *Acta Medica Scandinavica* Suppl. 1947; 196: 250.
5. Murray G, Delorme E, Thomas N. Artificial kidney. *Journal of the American Medical Association* 1948; 137: 1596.
6. Drukker W. Haemodialysis: a historical review. In: Drukker W, Parsons FM, Maher JF, eds. *Replacement of Renal Function by Dialysis*. The Hague: Martinus Nijhoff, 1978. Drukker learned from Tadeus Orlowski in 1977 that this kidney finally landed in the Jageliellonian University of Cracow, but that it was not used there, for lack of means.
7. Snapper invited Kolff to visit a number of university hospitals in the United States. One of the results was the first successful application of the artificial kidney in the United States. On this trip Kolff also visited the Peter Bent Brigham Hospital in Boston and there he met Dr Carl Walter, the head of the Fenwall Laboratories. He asked Kolff for the technical drawings of the rotating kidney and Kolff gave them and discussed a number of technical improvements. These were worked out by his co-worker Dr Olson. This was the origin of the 'Kolff–Brigham kidney', a version of which had some 40 specimens distributed later.

9

NEW WAYS OF FIGHTING URAEMIA

After the liberation papers appeared in some medical journals on other ways of treating renal patients. Kolff did not ignore them, but he applied these methods too, and compared the results with those of dialysis with the artificial kidney. He was interested primarily in the best way to treat patients with renal disease, not necessarily with a method he had developed himself.

In doing so he followed the example of Dr J. Mulder, the head of the clinic who was responsible under Professor Polak Daniels when Kolff had received his training in internal medicine in Groningen. Dr Mulder had invested much time and energy in attempts to develop vaccines and antisera against pneumonia – but as soon as sulphonamides came on the market he studied their value and very soon he preferred these above his own sera and vaccines. This meant that he referred his own studies of the preceding years to the archives.

9.1 PERITONEAL DIALYSIS

Kolff had already mentioned in his doctoral thesis the attempt by Rhoads in 1938 to use the patient's peritoneum as a dialysing membrane. Rhoads introduced about 10 litres of saline into the abdominal cavity and removed it again by suction some time later. An exchange of compounds had then taken place between the saline and the blood via the peritoneum. The fluid had to remain a long time in the peritoneal cavity to obtain a satisfactory delivery of urea and other compounds, and this increased the risk of peritonitis. In addition the water and salt balance was in danger of being disturbed if the composition of the saline solution had not been adapted sufficiently to the patient's needs.

At least four other authors reported the clinical application of this technique, now known as peritoneal dialysis. 'It is remarkable how widely spread in the medical literature of the world articles on the subject appeared and equally remarkable how little the various authors have been aware of each other's work, with the result that they have repeated the same experiments and the same mistakes', was Kolff's conclusion.[1]

Kolff thought that this treatment, now known as peritoneal dialysis, might become an alternative for treatment with the artificial kidney provided the rinsing fluid had a better composition and provided better precautions were taken against infection. This treatment might be useful for patients for whom heparin could not be used.

His assistant P. S. M. Kop applied peritoneal dialysis in the treatment of 21 patients in 1946 and 1947. Six of them were discharged with adequate renal function. They included two patients with bichloride of mercury intoxication, one (out of two) with a hepatorenal syndrome, one with symmetrical necrosis of the renal cortex, one with anuria due to renal calculi and one (out of two) with prostatic carcinoma with urethral obstruction. A full description is given in the thesis on which Kop obtained his doctorate in medicine at the University of Groningen in 1948. Professor Brinkman again acted as the promoter.[2]

Kolff and Kop concluded that peritoneal dialysis was an alternative that should be used sometimes instead of, or in combination with, haemodialysis.

9.2 INTESTINAL PERFUSION

The observation that vomiting and diarrhoea cause loss of urea led to attempts to make use of diarrhoea in the treatment of patients with uraemia. The results were disappointing.

Seligman, Frank and Fine concluded from experiments on dogs that the clearance of urea by 10 inches of jejunal loop was about 10% of normal renal function.[3]

This approach to the treatment of patients with uraemia was also tried out in Kampen. Kolff was assisted in this work in 1946 by Miss Nannie K. de Leeuw, an interne who had taken part in the development of the artificial kidney as a senior medical student in 1944. (She was to install an artificial kidney in Montreal in 1948, as will be described in a later chapter.)

Colonic perfusion through an appendix fistula was tried in two patients with severe hypertension and contracted kidneys, but the results were disappointing and this technique was abandoned.[4]

A double-ended ileostomy made an isolated loop of 1 m of terminal ileum accessible for perfusion in a patient with malignant hypertension and contracted kidneys. The best recovery was 5 grams of urea during a 10-hour perfusion, but this could not prevent a steady rise of his blood urea level. He returned home with equipment for intestinal perfusion. His wife nursed him with great care until his death two months later.[5]

This approach was continued in Kampen by E. E. Twiss, again under the guidance of Kolff. An intestinal loop of about 2 m was made in two patients. Another approach, made in nine patients, consisted of making the patient swallow a duodenal catheter. The duodenum was rinsed slowly via this catheter with a saline solution, collected in the rectum via a stiff tube. More details may be found in the thesis on which Twiss obtained his doctorate of medicine, Professor Brinkman acting as his promoter.[6]

At this time haemodialysis and peritoneal dialysis were only accessible only in a hospital; their application for patients with a chronic renal dysfunction raised many problems. Intestinal dialysis seemed to offer hope of becoming a technique that could be applied at home by such patients themselves at night, leaving them free to work in the daytime.

Since then haemodialysis and peritoneal lavage have become more accessible and safe. Hence it does not seem likely that the solution for renal problems will be sought further in development of intestinal lavage.

9.3 NON-ROTATING ARTIFICIAL KIDNEYS

The application of the rotating artificial kidney developed by Kolff may easily cause fluctuations in the patient's blood volume that would be life-threatening for children. Therefore one of the ways explored by Kolff was the development of a smaller non-rotating artificial kidney, suitable for use in children. In the meantime Alwall in Sweden[7] and Skeggs and Leonards in the USA[8] had described such compact machines. Gordon Murray in Toronto[9] also worked with such an apparatus.

Perspex and other kinds of plastic became available after World War II; they made it much easier to construct unorthodox apparatus, and so a simple apparatus could be built in Kampen, in which a cellophane tube was fixed flat in a channel through which rinsing fluid flowed. Blood flowed through the cellophane tube in a direction opposite to the one in which the rinsing fluid flowed (the countercurrent principle was applied here). Kolff named this apparatus after his first chemical technician, Mieneke van der Leij; the 'Mieneke model II' has found application in the Academic Hospital in Leiden (see Figure 9.1).

The power of this dialysing apparatus was much smaller than that of the rotating kidney; on the other hand it required much less supervision in operation. It could remain connected to the patient for a long time without any problem.

9.4 DIETARY REDUCTION OF PROTEIN BREAKDOWN

Due to frequent vomiting and anorexia, renal patients usually take up too little food to cover their energy needs. As a result the body breaks down more protein to obtain energy, resulting in an extra amount of nitrogenous waste products which such patients cannot excrete in their urine. Increasing the amount of carbohydrate (as sugar, for instance) and fat slows down the breakdown of protein for energy. That is the basis of the rice diet advised by Kempner in 1945 and of the low-protein carbohydrate and fat diet recommended by Professor Borst in the Netherlands.[10] This diet challenges the imagination of the patient and of the dietician to introduce variation in the otherwise monotonous flow of cooled butterballs coated with sugar.

Kolff added this diet to his arsenal of methods for the treatment of renal patients.

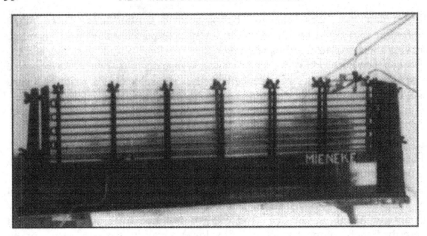

Figure 9.1 The non-rotating artificial kidney 'Mieneke'. Arterial blood is made to flow in a thin layer through a cellophane tube about 5 m long which is surrounded by rinsing fluid in an S-shaped channel; the fluid flows in a direction contrary to that of the blood (hence the principle of counter-current flow was incorporated in the design). The rinsing fluid flows through a channel in a series of plates of Perspex, a plastic material that became available only after the end of World War II. This type of kidney was developed by Kolff after 1945, a specimen has been used for some years in Leiden. However, the twin-coil kidney took its place soon after.

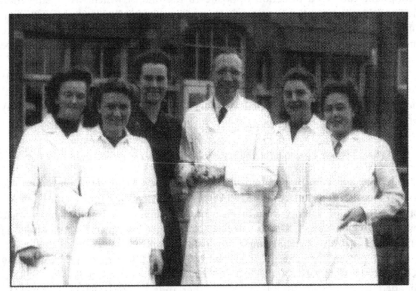

Figure 9.2 One of Kolff's claims for his appointment in Kampen in 1940 had been the appointment of a chemical technician. As a result Miss A. J. W. van der Leij was appointed. When she left to get married in 1947 there were five technicians working for Kolff. From left to right: Miss Wies Cley, Miss Truus Bakker, Miss Van der Leij, Miss Corrie Knol and Miss Willy Eskes.

His open attitude towards new methods as an alternative to treatment with the artificial kidney made it even more interesting to work with him; in fact he had no reason to complain of a lack of assistants. Not without a note of pride he could publish the results of his work with them in a combined text under the title *New Ways of Treating Uraemia.*[1]

All these experimental studies called for a great number of chemical analyses. Miss Mieneke van der Leij, his first technician whose appointment in 1941 had been one of Kolff's conditions for accepting an appointment in Kampen, left in 1947 to get married. By that time the number of technicians had increased to four (see Figure 9.2).

NOTES

1. Kolff WJ, with the cooperation of J. van Noordwijk, P. S. M. Kop, N. K. M. de Leeuw and A. M. Joekes. *New Ways of Treating Uraemia.* Londen: J & A Churchill, 1947.

2. Kop PSM. Peritoneaal dialyse (Peritoneal dialysis). Thesis for obtaining the doctorate in medicine at the University of Groningen on 7 July 1948. The promoter was Professor R. Brinkman. Kampen: J. H. Kok NV.

3. Seligman AM, Frank HA, Fine J. Treatment of experimental uremia by means of peritoneal irrigation. *Journal of Clinical Investigation* 1946; 25: 211.

4. See note 1 above, page 101.

5. See note 1 above, page 102.

6. Twiss EE. Treatment of uremia by dialysis and other methods with special regard to the principles and scope of intestinal dialysis. Thesis for the doctorate of medicine at the University of Groningen on 29 November 1950. The promoter was Professor R. Brinkman. Rotterdam: M. Wyt en Zonen. See also: Twiss EE, Kolf WJ. Treatment of uraemia by perfusion of isolated intestinal loop. *Journal of the American Medical Association* 1951; 146: 1019.

7. Alwall N. On the artificial kidney.I. Apparatus for dialysis of blood *in vivo. Acta Medica Scandinavica* 1947; 128: 317. See also: Alwall N, Norviit L. On the artificial kidney. II. The effectivity of the apparatus. *Acta Medica Scandinavica* (Suppl.) 1947; 196: 250.

8. Skeggs LT Jr, Leonards JR. Studies on an artificial kidney. I. Preliminary results with a new type of continuous dialyser. *Science* 1948; 108: 212. See also: Skeggs LT Jr, Leonards JR, Heisler CR. Artificial kidney. II. Construction and operation of an improved continuous dialyser. *Proceedings, Society for Experimental Biology and Medicine* 1949; 72: 539.

9. Murray G, Delorme E, Thomas N. Artificial kidney. *Journal of the American Medical Association* 1948; 137: 1596.

10. Borst JGG. Protein katabolism in uremia. Effects of protein-free diet, infections and blood transfusions. *Lancet* 1948; 1: 824.

10
BREATHING WITH A KIDNEY

On the morning after it had become clear that patient number 10 would survive his acute renal insufficiency after treatment with the artificial kidney Kolff said to me 'Now I know how you have to make the connections for an artificial heart.'

We had noticed in the very first dialysis on the first patient that the dark venous blood from the patient gradually became lighter as it passed through the coils of the cellophane tube; by the time it left the cellophane its colour was more like that of arterial blood.

It was clear that the power of the apparatus as an artificial lung was far too low to have any practical significance. To raise the capacity one would have to let much more blood flow through the apparatus, but it would not be easy to get so much blood out of an underarm or a leg. If one could solve that problem it would in fact result in a heart–lung machine! That was the problem Kolff thought he had solved after the treatment of the 10th patient.

For the time being there were no means and opportunities for experiments. When one of the professors of internal medicine was told by Kolff about his ideas after World War II he gave him a long incredulous look and said: 'But Mr Kolff, that is IMPOSSIBLE!' It was probably exactly the challenge Kolff needed to show that it was not.

A medical student, C. P. Dubbelman, started experimenting with a heart-lung machine some time after World War II in an empty garage of the hospital. To test the capacity, calves were used. Very useful assistance was given by the local Food Rationing Bureau: the number of heads of cattle awarded to the town of Kampen in that period was one higher than indicated by the size of the population, so that one could be used for Kolff's experiments first.

In 1949 the stage was reached that a calf could live for a quarter of an hour on the oxygen delivered by the heart–lung machine while its own lungs were shut off from the air. Kolff held his public lecture as a Reader at the University of Leiden in that year under the title: 'Life without heart and kidneys'. He described a patient in the future who would wear an artificial heart and artificial kidneys in a kind of backpack while his own heart and kidneys had been removed as useless non-functioning organs.

However, progress did not move that fast. Such a development called for much greater and longer lasting investments than the Netherlands could support at that time, impoverished and bereft as it was after World War II. Marshall Aid had only just started in 1947. The establishment of a communist regime in Czechoslovakia in 1948 meant that the Russian dictatorship had penetrated deeply into Central Europe. Kolff's family in the meantime had grown to five children. What kind of a future would they find in the Netherlands? Should they run the risk of growing up under a dictatorial regime?

On the other side of the Atlantic Ocean America was enticing: Kolff had been entertained there shortly before, on a tour with lectures on the artificial kidney that had become a real triumphal procession. Page and Corcoran did research on hypertension in Cleveland, and Kolff saw a great number of opportunities for research with the heart–lung machine.

All these considerations made Kolff decide to leave Kampen. He proposed Page to put his own knowledge of dialysis together with Page's knowledge of hypertension, and so bring the heart–lung machine to further development. Page agreed with this, and offered Kolff a position in his institute. Kolff accepted this offer.

The research in progress was rounded off. Dubbelman obtained his doctorate thesis on his work with the heart–lung machine; Professor Duyff in Leiden acted as his promoter.

After Kolff had left Kampen at the beginning of 1950 the development of the artificial kidney continued on the other side of the Atlantic Ocean – but at a much slower rate than Kolff had foreseen.

11

THE KIDNEY IN CANADA AND THE USA

11.1 THE ARTIFICIAL KIDNEY IN MONTREAL

In 1947 Kolff had sent one of the four kidneys he had built in Kampen shortly before the last winter of the war to the Royal Victoria Hospital in Montreal. Miss Nannie K. M. de Leeuw, a medical doctor who had taken part in the development of the artificial kidney with Kolff as a medical student in 1944 and as an interne in 1946, was given the opportunity to work with this kidney from 1948 on (see Figure 11.1). She received a scholarship from the Archibald Surgical Research Fund, under the direction of Dr G. Gavin Miller and Dr J. T. Maclean.

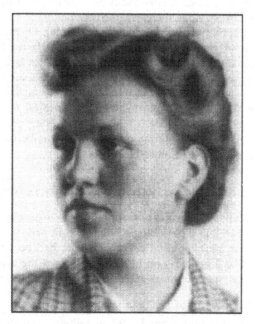

Figure 11.1 Miss Nannie K. M. de Leeuw: she worked with Kolff as a senior medical student and as a resident in 1946. In 1948 she installed a rotating kidney in the Royal Victoria Hospital in Montreal.

After her arrival in Montreal in February 1948 she had to start from scratch putting the kidney in working order in an environment to which she was completely unfamiliar.[1] That she succeeded in getting the kidney into action 11 days later (by way of speaking and literally) was therefore quite a remarkable achievement!

The first preliminary paper on this subject appeared in the same year;[2] it contained a brief description of the treatment of three patients. Kolff had mentioned an acute intoxication by an overdose of hypnotics as one of the indications for treatment with the kidney: such an overdose was indeed the reason for the treatment of the second patient in Montreal. Fortunately this treatment was successful.

A short while later she could report the treatment of three more patients.[3]

She had been interested for a long time in human blood cells. She used her time in Montreal to study the effect of dialysis with a rotating artificial kidney on the composition of blood.[4] It became clear that the number of leucocytes and platelets went down when a sample of blood passed through a cellophane tube on a rotating drum (the leucocytes stick to the cellophane tube). She confirmed the observation in Kampen, in 1943, that glycerine remaining in the cellophane tube may damage the erythrocytes. A new observation was that the roller pump may also damage the erythrocytes.

There was yet another artificial kidney in Montreal. Dr M. Korenberg had a kidney built himself in the Jewish General Hospital, based on the drawings in Kolff's doctoral thesis. He had introduced some improvements, but unfortunately contacts between the two kidney teams were too scarce to spread these improvements.

One year later the urology department of the hospital took charge of the kidney. By the time Kolff could see it himself, much later, the twin-coil kidney had been developed and the rotating drum kidney was becoming a historical monument in a museum (see Figure 11.2).

11.2 THE ARTIFICIAL KIDNEY IN LONDON, ONTARIO

In this case it was not an internist or a surgeon who organized the installation of an artificial kidney, but a physiologist interested in peripheral blood flow in humans. The British physiologist Dr Otto Edholm had become familiar with the work of Kolff, in England, and he came to regard the artificial kidney as an instrument that would make interesting experimental medical studies possible.

He was appointed to the chair of physiology at the University of Western Ontario in London, Ontario, Canada. When Edholm heard from Kolff that I was working in Toronto at that time, but would terminate work there in the middle of 1948, he asked whether I would be willing to come to London, Ontario.[5] Edholm obtained the cooperation of Dr Brien and Dr Watson, the professors of internal medicine and of clinical pathology respectively at the

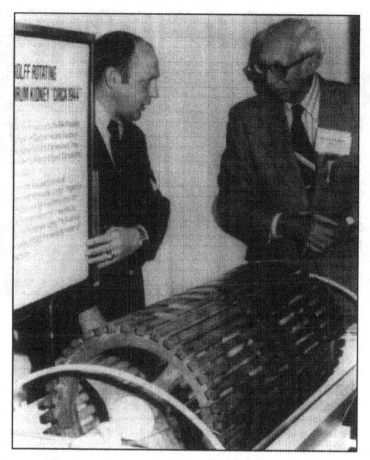

Figure 11.2 P. T. McBride, the director of the firm of Baxter that produced 'twin-coil kidneys', and Kolff again examined the rotating kidney in Montreal that Miss Nannie K. M. de Leeuw installed there in 1948.

University of Western Ontario. He succeeded in collecting the funds needed to build a kidney from the drawings in Kolff's doctoral thesis, and to let me work for a year in London, Ontario.

I arrived there with my wife at the end of August 1948. Dr Edholm's department of physiology was housed in the Medical School and the kidney was built there in the workshop of the technician Mr Allingham. As shown in Figure 11.3 it was of the classical rotating type.

The press service of the university saw to it that a reporter came to interview me when the kidney was ready. At that time contact with the press was one of the heaviest sins that a medical doctor could commit, according to the current medical ethics. However, the New World had a completely different opinion

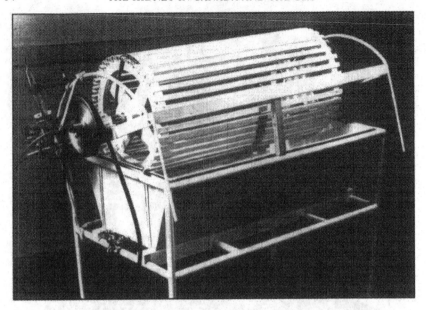

Figure 11.3 The rotating artificial kidney that the author installed in London (Ontario) and used for his study on the role of phenols in acute renal insufficiency. The cylinder has been tilted to make it easier to clean the tank.

about publicity, and that was something I had not realized sufficiently. Directly after a photograph of the kidney with me bending over it had appeared in the daily paper I was phoned by a furious Mr Allingham because I had omitted to mention his name as the builder of the kidney! The idea that he suggested that he was the spiritual father of the machine infuriated me in turn. After a hell of a row we had cleared the air and we were able to make peace again.

The kidney was installed in the Medical School; this building was connected to the Royal Victoria Hospital by a tunnel, so that the kidney could be transported quickly to the hospital when needed for the treatment of a patient. Apart from this it was available for the experimental research which I had planned in consultation with Dr Edholm and Dr Rossiter, the professor of biochemistry.

The object of that study was the group of compounds accumulating in renal insufficiency. Studies at the beginning of the 19th century had indicated that this causes an accumulation of several organic compounds having in common a phenol group. Other studies had shown that many of these phenolic compounds cause drowsiness. Hence the drowsiness observed in many renal patients was ascribed to accumulation of such phenolic compounds. However, shortly after World War II many new methods were developed for measuring the concentration of a compound in blood or urine, based on other principles. It became clear that the classical methods were often less specific than the technician expected, and that the real concentration of the compound to be measured was much lower than the classical method indicated. To discover whether this would also apply to phenolic compounds in renal failure we did a short series of experiments on dogs. Briefly, the result was that blocking renal excretion in dogs over a period of one to four days did not lead to an important accumulation of phenols. Hence we concluded that phenolic compounds play at the most a minor role in acute renal failure.

Meanwhile the kidney was used for a patient with acute anuria after an operation. He was treated once, and after that his renal function recovered so that he was discharged in good health from the hospital.

In July 1949 I handed over the care of the artificial kidney to one of the co-workers of Dr Watson, and I returned to the Netherlands with my family.

That kidney had a quiet old age. Edholm, who had gone back to England at the beginning of 1949, returned to London, Ontario, some years later, and asked what had been done with the kidney. It was stored in a cupboard under a sheet – nicely cleaned, but not in use.

11.3 SIRE OF 'KIDNEY' IS FRANKFURTER: A LEECH ALSO HELPED

I am sure Kolff never described the kidney in these terms, but they were used in the *Milwaukee Journal* of 24 November 1949 to introduce the story of the first successful application of the kidney in Columbia Hospital in Milwaukee.

Less than a year earlier one of the employees of the Allis–Chalmers Manufacturing Company in Milwaukee was struck down by a renal disease. When the directors realized that no artificial kidney was available for his treatment they decided to present one to the city of Milwaukee. They sent one of their engineers on a mission to Dr Palmer in Vancouver, to Dr Merrill in Boston, and to me in London, Ontario, to look at the rotating artificial kidneys there with a technical eye. He also went to Dr Gordon Murray in Toronto who had developed a non-rotating type of artificial kidney. After comparing the engineer's reports the firm decided to take the kidney in London, Ontario, as their model. Early in the spring of 1949 I was invited to come and see the result. It had been tested rigorously: it had rotated continuously for 24 hours, monitored by engineers on an eight-hour shift! It was a beauty and I said spontaneously that this was the kidney we had been dreaming of when we built ours in Kampen during the war! The reaction was a request right away to address all the employees of the factory who had taken part in building it, and tell them the story of the development in Kampen! I did so. It really was a magnificent apparatus, with all the improvements I had suggested to the engineer who saw the kidney in London, Ontario. One of these was a Perspex hood over the rotating drum to prevent the evaporation of fluid and to muffle the noise.

On 25 July I was in Toronto with my wife and five-week-old son on our way back to the Netherlands, when I received a phone call to come to Milwaukee for the first application of the kidney. I had no visa for the USA, and getting one had taken me at least two months, before. However, they called the American consul in his summer cottage and I had a visa within two hours, in time for the plane to Milwaukee! By Tuesday afternoon it was clear that the patient's kidney function had recovered spontaneously, the application was cancelled and I flew back to London, Ontario, in time to do the final oral examination for my MSc thesis on Wednesday afternoon and to catch the train to Toronto that evening. We sailed back to the Netherlands from Montreal a week later.

Twice more the application of that kidney was called off at the last moment, but on 21 November 1949 the kidney made by Allis–Chalmers was indeed used, as reported in the *Milwaukee Journal*. The patient was a 55-year-old man from Michigan with an acute nephritis due to an allergic reaction. His kidneys had failed for the preceding five days. Before the reader of the *Milwaukee Journal* gets to the description of the procedure he is reminded discreetly that the kidney had been donated to the community by the Allis–Chalmers Manufacturing Company, which had taken months in developing it at a cost of $10 000. A three-hour dialysis was performed by a team trained in Boston (see Figure 11.4). Two days later the patient's kidneys had resumed their function again so that he could return home (see Figure 11.5). This first application of the kidney was seen as 'a success beyond our greatest hopes' by the doctors monitoring the operation.

This newspaper report states at the end that knowledge of the design of the machine was gained by correspondence with its inventor, Dr W. J. Kolff of Amsterdam, Holland. An anonymous contributor donated a second kidney (at a cost of $4500) to the Marquette University medical school for use at the county hospital. The reporter learned that it was to be tried on dogs next week and was expected to be used on a human patient a week later.

A third machine built by Allis–Chalmers was to be shipped to Cleveland, Ohio, to be used by Dr Irvin Page. In fact it was there when Kolff arrived in Cleveland in 1950. (It had cost about $5600; Kolff concluded that it worked just as well as the kidneys that had cost about $200 each in Kampen.)

An even more exciting report appeared in the *Milwaukee Journal* of 8 December 1949. A 57-year-old man had received a blood transfusion for bleeding stomach ulcers, but the blood given was incompatible with his own and the result was an acute renal failure. When this had lasted eight days he was connected to the artificial kidney of the county hospital, which had been rushed to St Joseph's general hospital for this occasion. By the time the patient was wheeled into the operating room he was unconscious and his breathing was irregular; the injection of the local anaesthetic to introduce a cannula into a left arm artery caused no reaction. Twenty minutes after the dialysis started the patient began to take notice of his surroundings; three hours and 15 minutes later he was alert and answered questions.

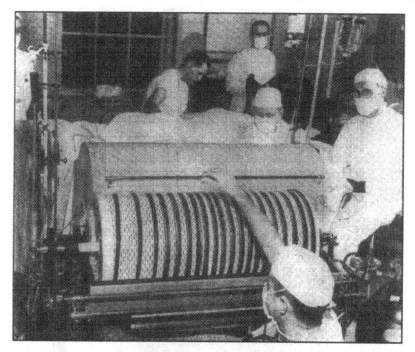

Figure 11.4 The application of the artificial kidney built by Allis-Chalmers in Milwaukee on the first patient, November 1949. The hood covering the cylinder has been raised to inspect the cellophane tube.

This dialysis was monitored by a team of five young county hospital residents, who had tried out the kidney on dogs: we can only hope that the experience gained with the application of the kidney before on at least 20 human patients by that time in Kampen, The Hague, Amsterdam, Montreal and London (Ontario) was used. Three scientists from Allis–Chalmers were on hand to see that the apparatus run smoothly. About fifty doctors, nurses, technicians and sisters watched the dialysis, which lasted two hours and 40 minutes.

As the patient returned to his room, where relatives had gathered in prayer with a minister during the time he was away, he was breathing well, his blood pressure was normal, his pulse was good and his mind clear and active. He continued to improve the next day.

According to the *Milwaukee Journal* of 24 November 1949 the Allis–Chalmers Manufacturing Company had been asked by 25 hospitals whether they would continue to manufacture such machines. Allis–Chalmers did in fact supply 14 of these kidneys to several hospitals in the United States, *inter alia* in Los Angeles. However, the firm discontinued this project at the beginning of the 1950s because of lack of interest from clinicians.

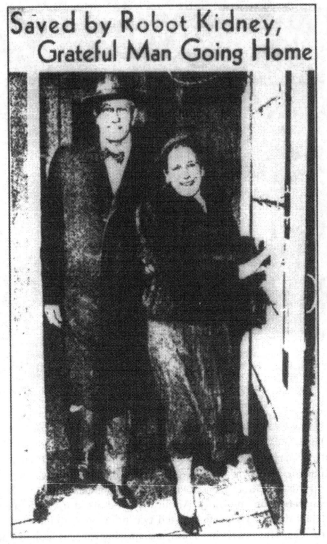

Figure 11.5 'Fate stepped in to get me here' said the first patient treated with the artificial kidney in Milwaukee on going home two weeks after his dialysis.

What was the reason that the artificial kidney was introduced in some clinics, but not used very much?

Patients for whom treatment with the kidney was indicated only came in very irregularly, but such treatment did demand the availability of a whole team of doctors, nurses and chemical technicians. These artificial kidneys do

not work without the constant attention of someone who has sufficient authority to press the application on a patient in spite of technical and organizational
difficulties. The rotating kidney remained in use only under the guidance of a
person who was convinced that this apparatus offered possibilities that could
not be realized in any other way.

11.4 FRUSTRATION IN CLEVELAND

A simple non-rotating artificial kidney had been developed by Skeggs and
Leonards in Cleveland, Ohio[6] while Kolff was still in Kampen. They used
sheets of cellophane clamped between two grooved rubber plates. Blood flowed
through the grooves on one side of the cellophane, a rinsing fluid through the
grooves in the other rubber plate. Cleveland was also the place where Corcoran
and Page worked, well known from their studies of hypertension. That was
the reason that Kolff had contacted Page from the Netherlands, as described
above.

Page responded and gave Kolff a post in his clinic. However, after Kolff had
emigrated to Cleveland with his family Page proved to have had quite another
goal in attracting Kolff: he made clear that he expected Kolff to support him
in his own research. He had very little interest in the artificial kidney and even
less in the heart–lung machine. Neither did the surgeons in the Cleveland Clinic
show any interest at that time in a heart–lung machine. There was nothing left
for Kolff but to put his apparatus in a cupboard and hope that better times
would come.

Fortunately Janke Kolff supported her husband staunchly in those difficult
years in Cleveland. She had supported him in the difficult war years in Kampen
by seeing to it that there was always food on the table, not only for their
children but also for the unexpected guest. This was a task that called for quite
a bit of manoeuvring as food rationing became more severe all the time.

In Cleveland Janke continued to keep up spirits during the seven years that
elapsed there before Kolff had built up what he had left behind in Kampen.
He felt that he was thrown back from a very productive life to a non-productive
existence. Kolff and Janke had five children, no household help, and very little
money. That Janke helped to think up ways of enjoying life in that period is
something for which Kolff openly expressed his admiration. The only type of
holiday they could afford was to go camping – and they enjoyed it.[7]

11.5 THE TWIN-COIL KIDNEY, SUITABLE FOR MASS PRODUCTION

Better times seemed to begin in 1955 when an Austrian doctor, Dr Bruno
Watschinger, came to Cleveland.

In the early 1950s Watschinger had become interested in the renal function
of rats used for the study of hypertension.[8] He became involved in the determination of the renal clearance of several compounds in a number of diseases

including hypertension. For that reason he applied for a WHO grant for a research fellowship to study renal disease. However, one day his chief decided that he should not become a nephrologist but a rheumatologist, because he needed one for his department. Fortunately his chief changed his opinion again shortly after, so Watschinger could pursue his original plan and try to become a nephrologist.

Watschinger stated three arguments for preferring a stay at the Cleveland Clinic: it was the place where Dr Page worked – at that time a guru in the field of hypertension, also Dr Corcoran and Dr Henriette Duston, specialists when it came to measuring renal clearance, and also Dr Kolff, the man of the famous rotating kidney and other methods for the treatment of renal diseases.

Shortly after his arrival in the Cleveland Clinic, and the traditional cup of tea with Kolff, Watschinger was required to measure the clotting time every 15 minutes in a patient who was being treated for an acute renal disturbance. Of course it was nice to see the famous rotating kidney in action, but this was not the kind of research he had in mind. It would be much more valuable for him to become familiar with new methods for renal research that were being applied in other sections of the Cleveland Clinic. Not a single medical organization in postwar Austria had the financial means to use such an expensive rotating kidney. Kolff asked him repeatedly to spend the full three months of his grant in his department – but Watschinger said no: he failed to see how on earth he would be able to import the rotating kidney into Austria. The thing Vienna needed was a cheap dialysing apparatus with low running costs that needed only few technically trained people in application. This argument Kolff countered by saying 'Okay, let's make one that can be used easily.' He added that he would try to get money to let Watschinger stay for a longer period. Watschinger hesitated: at that time Kolff was engaged in a project with cardiac surgeons to improve the oxygen supply in open-heart operations. In addition Kolff no longer showed much interest in the kidney. However, this conversation brought his interest to life again, and he convinced Watschinger that his experience with dialysing machines would be extremely valuable in the development of a simple, cheap kidney. Still Watschinger hesitated; he had promised his wife, who could not come with him to Cleveland, that he would be home again after three months.

But Fate smiled at him, assuming the face of his wife: she convinced him that, never mind his promise, he should stay with Kolff – something to which he paid tribute to her in his report of this study.[8]

At that time the only other type of artificial kidney in use, in addition to Kolff's rotating kidney, was the plate dialyser designed by Skeggs and Leonards. In 1953 a group of surgeons led by Inouye and Engelberg[9] had described a simple artificial kidney, in which blood flowed through a cellophane tube submerged in a pressure cooker. As the rinsing fluid in the pressure cooker was housed in a closed system, not only dialysis but also ultrafiltration could take place as long as the pressure in the rinsing fluid differed from that in the blood. However, this concept of using a pressure difference between blood and rinsing fluid gained little support, and the authors themselves did not continue work in this direction either.

Nevertheless Kolff and Watschinger were attracted by the idea of a roll of cellophane tube with a separation between the different windings. They used a cheap, mass-produced, glass-fibre fly screen to separate the windings: this material was on the market to keep flies out of a stable. Strips of this fly screen also served to keep the correct distance between the two layers of fly screen enclosing the cellophane tube, so that an optimal ratio between the blood flow and the surface of the cellophane tube would be maintained. Their experiments indicated that a cushion of two layers of fly screen was optimal. The next problem then came their way: if they rolled the cellophane tube with the fly screen on both sides of it by hand it was hard to do it under a constant tension – and when the tension changed the blood flow through the cellophane tube changed too! Kolff developed a simple solution in the basement of his home: he used some wood and empty cans to build a simple machine to wind the cellophane tube and its screens under constant tension.

They tried first to fix the two layers of fly screen and the cushion of fly screen between them with cement, but that was not satisfactory. An employee from a clothing factory helped them out: he sewed the layers together with his sewing machine (see Figure 11.6). That solution brought them to the last

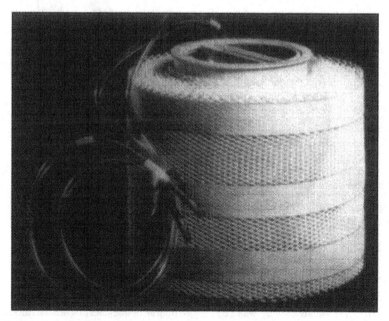

Figure 11.6 One of the first versions of the 'twin-coil kidney' of Kolff and Watschinger.

problem: what do you use as the kernel for the role of cellophane tube plus screen? One day, during lunch, their eyes fell on a heap of empty cans: that was it! They tried empty beer cans, small and large fruit-juice cans. Watschinger measured the clearance every time in such an apparatus – an empty pineapple juice can with 10 m of cellophane tube proved to be the best combination. The small beer cans gave too high a resistance. Finally they laid a second cellophane tube of 10 m alongside the first one to double the capacity – hence the name 'twin-coil kidney' (see Figure 11.7).

This apparatus was presented at a scientific congress in 1955. Kolff's 'research' section produced and sterilized a series of these apparatuses for clinical use; in 1956 they were able to publish the encouraging results of 11 dialyses in eight patients.[10]

This twin-coil kidney signified a breakthrough in two respects: it gave renal patients and nephrologists reason to hope that they too would shortly have a simple dialysing apparatus at their disposal. The way was opened for the medical industry to start the mass production of a dialysing apparatus as a

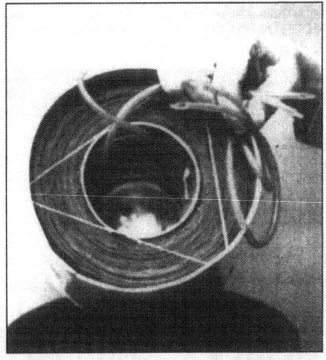

Figure 11.7 The 'twin-coil kidney' with a core copied from an orange-juice can: hence its nickname 'orange-juice kidney'.

disposable article for which all the necessary ingredients were available on the market at a low price. The pump needed for this apparatus was simple to make.

As a matter of fact the mass production proved not to be so easy to launch: the development of this kidney in Kolff's department had taken three weeks, but it took five months before Kolff had found a firm willing to start production. However, before long at least 500 of these kidneys had been delivered to clinics in the United States.[13]

11.6 THE ARTIFICIAL KIDNEY IN BOSTON

Kolff's American tour in 1947 had included the Peter Bent Brigham Hospital in Boston, at the invitation of Dr George Thorn of the Harvard Medical School. At that moment Kolff had no more artificial kidneys available to give away, so he gave Dr C. Walter copies of the drawings from his doctoral thesis.

These copies enabled Dr Edward Olsen, an engineer working with Dr Walter, to build a kidney essentially identical with the kidneys from Kampen, but enriched with the refinements that were made possible financially and technically in the United States at that time (see Figure 11.8).

This so-called 'Kolff–Brigham kidney' was used for the first time for a patient on 11 June 1948. In the following 15 years Dr Olsen delivered another 40 specimens of this kidney: they went *inter alia* to Switzerland, the United Kingdom, Italy, France, Belgium, Argentina, Brazil, Chile, Uruguay, Venezuela, Costa Rica, Mexico and Japan. A new development was the formation of a kidney team in Boston under the direction of the surgeon Dr Charles Hufnagel and the internist Dr John P. Merrill (see Figure 11.9).

Dr Merrill's original interest was not kidney disease but heart disease, especially the effect of electrolyte changes on the electrocardiogram.[11] His first conclusion after looking at the kidney was that there must be a simpler way of taking over the function of the kidney – but the Professor of Hydraulic Engineering at MIT, whom he consulted, reported that he could think of no better way to do the job, as long as blood had to be used!

The very first patient they treated was a chronic uraemic, who had been comatose and convulsing for several days. The results of the three-hour dialysis were disappointing. It was only two days later that he improved so much that he started to sit up in bed, reading the comics over breakfast. Only much later Merrill realized that, in a patient who has been decompensated over some years, not all the abnormal blood chemistries can be restored to normal at once.

Merrill's interest in electrolytes and in the electrocardiogram founded a new field of study. The experience with the dialysis of potassium-intoxicated patients enabled his group to publish the first description of potassium intoxication and its reversal by dialysis. They also found that they could produce digitalis intoxication in digitalized patients simply by lowering their serum potassium level by dialysis.

A novel application of the ability to influence the electrolyte balance with

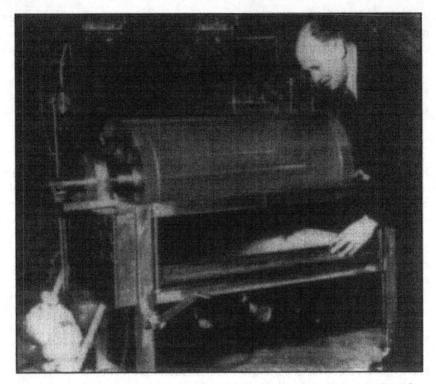

Figure 11.8 Mr Edward Olsen with the 'Kolff–Brigham kidney' developed at the Peter Bent Brigham Hospital in Boston.

dialysis was developed during the war in Korea for the treatment of wounded soldiers. This was the first war in which casualties could be transported rapidly to a field hospital by helicopter. They were often in shock so that their kidneys could not cope with the tissue breakdown products from their wounds. The result was often an acute potassium intoxication, endangering the heart. A Kolff–Brigham kidney was sent to Korea. Dr P. E. Teschan, a member of the surgical research team, wrote to Dr Olsen in November 1952 that the kidney worked just as well in the sawahs of Korea as in Washington, that they had carried out on average one dialysis per day since 11 October, and that at least 20 soldiers owed their life to this treatment[12] (see Figure 11.10). The drum of the kidney was fitted with a large crank for use under these circumstances, so that it could be revolved by hand in case there were a power break! Figure 11.11 shows the kidney in use in a field hospital.

Teschan probably did not realize that he described an effective solution for the medical problem which had made such a deep impression on Georg Haas during World War I, and which had induced him to attempt to develop an artificial kidney.

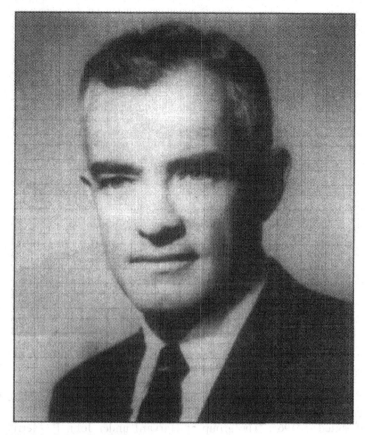

Figure 11.9 John P. Merrill, MD; he developed the use of the artificial kidney in Boston to a firm base for launching renal transplantation from 1963 onwards.

When Kolff and Watschinger had developed the 'twin-coil kidney' this was adopted rapidly by the Boston group. In 1964 this group started a programme for home dialysis.

Renal transplantations too were carried out in Boston as early as 1956. 'Many people from the transplantation field do not realize that it was our version of Kolff's artificial kidney which made the first transplantation possible', was Merrill's conclusion in 1984.[11] Merrill and the surgeon Dr Joseph Murray successfully transplanted kidneys at a time when the surgeons in Cleveland were still opposed to this. This opened new futures for patients with chronic renal failure: it encouraged spending time, effort and funds in dialysing them until a suitable donor kidney became available.

Apart from that, the presence of an efficiently working team attracted patients with acute renal failure from all over the world, and this made it possible for

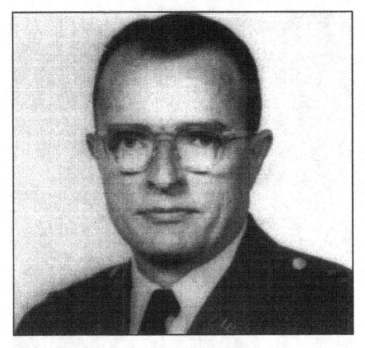

Figure 11.10   Paul Teschan, MD; after being trained in Boston by John Merrill he applied the artificial kidney at the 11th Evacuation Hospital in Korea.

Merrill and his group to study the clinical course of acute renal failure from many causes before and after dialysis.

Kolff stated in 1965: 'The group at Harvard under John P. Merrill have promoted the acceptance of dialysis more than any other group.'[13]

11.7   THE DEPARTMENT OF ARTIFICIAL ORGANS AT THE UNIVERSITY OF UTAH

Many surgeons at that time began to realize that their technique of heart surgery had several disadvantages. Kolff took his heart–lung machine out of the cupboard and resumed work on it. He managed to get an appointment both in the department of surgery and in the department of developmental research. When a new idea or a new programme was blocked in one department he transferred it to the other one, so he could often go on with it. But then the day arrived in 1967 when he was made to understand that he had to limit himself to one department. From the evening of that day on Kolff began to look out for another place to work.

He concluded that the University of Utah in Salt Lake City had one of the best regional medical programmes in the United States. When he became

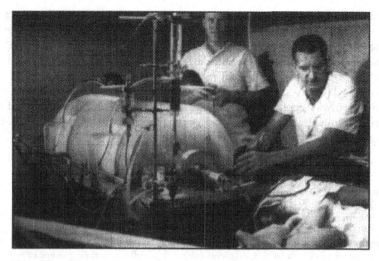

Figure 11.11 'You will be interested to know that the kidney works as well in a rice paddy in Korea as in Washington. ... Since 11 October we have averaged one dialysis per day and the patient influx continues', Paul Teschan wrote to Edward Olsen on 4 November 1952. This picture was taken in the 11th Evacuation Hospital in Korea.

convinced that he would obtain enough cooperation from the surgical department there, and that the university bureaucracy would interfere very little with his efforts to obtain funds, he began to regard that as the best place for carrying out his programme of artificial organs. He accepted an appointment as professor of surgery in the medical faculty and hence head of a department of artificial organs. In addition he was also appointed to the 'College of Engineering' (in the Faculty of Technical Sciences) as a professor for research, and as a consequence head of the Institute for Biomedical Technique.

In Utah, too, Kolff had to apply what has been called his almost 'alchemistical capacity to transform catastrophes into success'. Kolff himself remarked once that 'calamities and disasters have brought me advantages in the long run'.[14]

Under the worst conditions one can imagine he had organized the first blood bank on the continent of Europe in May 1940, and it is still functioning. He developed the artificial kidney during the German occupation of his country. In spite of all opposition he managed to improve the artificial kidney in Cleveland and to make progress with his heart–lung machine. He encountered much more cooperation in Utah, but nevertheless he was not spared setbacks, although they were of a different kind:

• A large number of sheep which he had bought for the development of the artificial heart were stolen. Obtaining funds for research in the following year had disappointing results – but then the insurance paid the compensation for the stolen sheep, and with that money Kolff could go on.

- In 1973 his laboratory burned down and could not be replaced. By renovating an old set of buildings of a local hospital Kolff and his co-workers obtained one of the most advanced laboratories for artificial organs of that period.
- The National Institutes of Health in Bethesda, the largest American institute for the organization of medical research, refused to grant permission to the group in Utah to implant an artificial heart in a human being – but then the American Secretary of Health delegated the decision to the Food and Drug Administration, and that adopted a more favourable standpoint with regard to this proposal.

NOTES

1. De Leeuw NKM. Personal communication.
2. MacLean JT, Ripstein CVB, de Leeuw NKM, Gavin Miller G. The use of the artificial kidney in the treatment of uraemia (Preliminary report). *Canadian Medical Association Journal* 1948; 58: 433–436. Patient 1 was in a very bad condition at the beginning of the dialysis and died a few hours after a dialysis of three hours. Patient 2 had taken a high dose of a hypnotic causing the production of urine to stop. His diuresis started again after a short dialysis and he recovered. Patient 3, a woman of 55 years with a bilateral closure of the urinary tract (probably on the basis of a congenital abnormality), came in in a bad condition due to a urinary tract infection. She was dialysed for six hours and her condition improved, her diuresis increased again and she left the hospital in a reasonable condition.
3. Ripstein CB, MacLean JT, de Leeuw NKM, Gavin Miller G. Clinical experiences with the artificial kidney. *Surgery* 1949; 26: 229–236. The fourth patient was a man of 20 years with polycystic kidneys who was dying when he came in. His condition improved so much after a dialysis of six hours that he could resume work after 10 days. Patient 5 was a man of 27 years with chronic nephritis who improved for a short time but he died 12 days after the dialysis. Anuria developed in patient 6 after an operation; his condition improved after a dialysis of six hours.
4. De Leeuw NKM, Blaustein A. Studies of blood passed through an artificial kidney. *Blood, the Journal of Hematology* 1949; 4: 653–666.
5. Noordwijk J van. Early history in Canada. *Dialysis and Transplantation* 1982; 11: 38. Kolff had distributed copies of the short English version of his doctoral thesis to all authors he had quoted and who were still alive. One of these was Dr D. Y. Solandt in Toronto: together with Thalhimer and Best he had described a dialysis on dogs with the use of heparin and cellophane. Solandt appreciated this very highly, and offered a starting post in research for young persons whom Kolff would consider suitable. Kolff suggested my name – and that is how I arrived in Toronto in August 1947 shortly after obtaining my physicians' licence in Groningen. My wife had obtained a position as a research assistant at the Banting and Best Institute in Toronto; her contribution to the study of the metabolism of animals with experimental diabetes mellitus she could use later, after our return to the Netherlands, as her minor in biochemistry for her master's degree in biology.

   Dr Solandt carried out research on the changes in skeletal muscle deprived of stimuli via its nerve, and my research was part of that study. Unfortunately Solandt was so much occupied by a large number of committees that he did not appear in the department for days on end. Sometimes he came in during the night – we noticed that because he left notes with news and directions in all kinds of places. That was not very stimulating.

   Toronto at that time impressed us as a weak infusion of an American city with the emphasis on the power of the dollar, and only a very light accent on cultural values. Although we had made close ties of friendship with a small number of Canadians we decided to go back to Europe in 1948. However, before doing so I was asked by Dr Edholm whether I was interested in installing an artificial kidney at the University of Western Ontario, for clinical application and experimental research. The atmosphere in London, Ontario, where that university was located was more provincial but very much more comradely.

6. Skeggs LT Jr, Leonards JR. Studies on an artificial kidney: I. Preliminary results with a new type of continuous dialyzer. *Science* 1948; 108: 212–213. See also Skeggs LT Jr, Leonards JR, Heisler CR. Artificial kidney. II. Construction and operation of an improved continuous dialyser. *Proceedings, Society for Experimental Biology and Medicine* 1949; 72: 539.
7. Kolff told this in the NOS television programme broadcast in February 1989 as part of the programme series 'Markant'.
8. Watschinger B. From the rotating drum to the pineapple-can coil kidney: the unpublished history of the twin-coil. *Artificial Organs* 1995; 9: 870–876.
9. Inouye WY and Engelberg J. A simplified artificial dialyzer and ultrafilter. *Surgical Forum* 1953; 4: 438–442.
10. Kolff WJ, Watschinger B, Vertes V. Results in patients treated with the coil kidney (disposable dialyzing unit). *Journal of the American Medical Association* 1956; 161: 1433–1437.
11. Merrill JP. The legacy of 'Pim' Kolff. *Nephron* 1984; 36: 153–155.
12. Teschan PE (cited by McBride PT) *Genesis of the Artificial Kidney*. Baxter Health Care Corporation, 1987.
13. Kolff WJ. First clinical experience with the artificial kidney. *Annals of Internal Medicine* 1965; 62: 608–619.
14. Weisse AB. Turning bad luck into good: the alchemy of Willem Johan Kolff. *Seminars in Dialysis* 1993; 6: 52–58.

THE PLACE OF THE ARTIFICIAL KIDNEY IN PRESENT-DAY MEDICINE – AND HOW IT WAS ACHIEVED

The artificial kidney is generally accepted now as an apparatus for chronic renal patients. It can help them get over a life-threatening renal dysfunction and it can offer them a life as nearly normal as possible, so long as they cannot get a kidney transplant. In addition it can be of help in acute intoxications.

More than half a million people all over the world were being dialysed regularly by the end of 1992. Haemodialysis with an artificial kidney was used by about 82% of them; the other 18% used peritoneal lavage.[1]

The development of the 'twin-coil kidney' was an important milestone on the road to the present position of the kidney: it was the first kidney that lent itself to mass production, making use of cheap, readily obtainable materials.

The following six factors influenced the way in which the present position was attained:

- industry's interest in the production;
- familiarity of the medical profession with this treatment;
- the accessibility of the patient's blood vessels;
- the possibility of dialysis at home;
- the development of renal transplantation;
- rulings for meeting the financial costs.

These factors influenced each other: the road opened by a development in one aspect sometimes became a cul-de-sac, or narrowed down to a footpath, until a development in another field – sometimes in a slightly different direction – opened the road up again. For this reason the historian gets a clear view of the development only if he keeps six eyes open at the same time, or in any case immediately pays attention to the other aspects when he has observed a development in one particular field.

Kidneys had been built in series on a small scale before the 'twin-coil kidney' was developed. Kolff himself had a series of four rotating kidneys built in Kampen. On arrival in Cleveland in 1950 he found a kidney built by Allis–Chalmers. This firm built a total of 14 kidneys but then lost interest in the product. The kidney built in Boston for the Peter Bent Brigham Hospital by Olsen on the basis of Kolff's drawings has become known as the 'Kolff–Brigham kidney'; some 40 specimens have spread out all over the world.

Two efforts by Kolff to arouse a manufacturer's interest for the production of the 'twin-coil kidney' were unsuccessful until he met Dr William B. Graham of the firm of Travenol, later the senior Chairman of the Baxter Health Corporation. Dr Graham, being a chemist, was familiar with the notions of diffusion and dialysis, and he realized the importance of this development. It did not take long before 500 specimens of the 'twin-coil kidney' had been delivered as disposable kidneys for single use at a price of $59; the matching bath for the rinsing fluid and the pump that could be used every time together cost $1080.

However, it soon turned out that very many apparatuses remained unused because only a few doctors were so familiar with the idea of dialysis as a way of treatment that they thought of resorting to the 'twin-coil kidney' at a time when this was a realistic option for one of their patients.

To stimulate its application in cases of acute intoxication Dr George Schreiner and Dr John Maher from the George Washington University in Washington, DC, developed standard operating procedures for the application in several acute intoxications, such as those resulting from an overdose of aspirin and other derivatives of salicylic acid. Dr Joseph Holmes organized courses on similar subjects at the University of Colorado.

These efforts were successful: the number of patients using the kidney rose, and dialysis was being accepted more and more as a way of treatment in acute temporary renal failure. But then the next obstacle arose: access to the patient's blood vessels when dialysis had to be repeated.

12.1 THE ACCESSIBILITY OF THE PATIENT'S BLOOD VESSELS FOR REPEATED DIALYSIS

An impetus to improving the access to blood vessels for repeated dialyses had already been given by P. E. Teschan[2] during the Korean war. He had introduced thin plastic tubes filled with saline and heparin into an artery and a vein. This made it possible to connect the same patient a number of times with an artificial kidney. However, clotting in the cannulae occurred a number of times, so this technique was discarded again.

W. E. Quinton and B. H. Scribner (Figure 12.1) developed another solution in Seattle in 1960. They introduced Teflon tubes into an artery and a vein; Teflon is a synthetic material to which fluids do not adhere. The Teflon tubes were pushed through the skin and connected with each other when they were not being used for a dialysis.[3] They used this technique on a patient on 9 March 1960 and dialysed him repeatedly (see Figure 12.2). Unfortunately failures occurred nevertheless: the stiff Teflon cannulae sometimes damaged the vessel wall, and the place where they penetrated the skin sometimes became infected.

In the following year they described an improved technique: Teflon was only used for the cannulae in the blood vessels, and they were connected by a silicone rubber tube that passed through the skin and was used for connecting

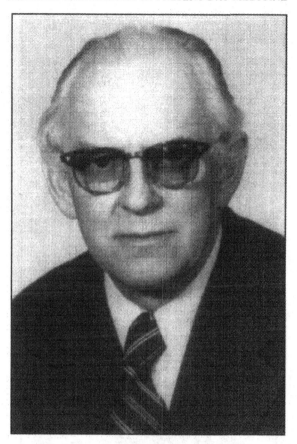

Figure 12.1 Belding Scribner, MD. With Wayne Quinton he developed the shunt (named after them) which greatly facilitated repeated dialyses of the same patient.

with the kidney.[4] That decreased the risk of leakage from the blood vessels – but the risk of infection remained.

A solution for this problem came from another direction in 1962. J. E. Cimino had learnt as a medical student that he could increase the blood flow from a vein by applying a blood pressure cuff to that vein (see Figure 12.3). Using a similar technique he succeeded in drawing enough blood from an underarm vein for the kidney without using an artery.[5] After the dialysis the needle was withdrawn from the vein, so no tube was left sticking through the skin and the risk of infection was diminished. In 1966 he and his co-workers described another improvement: the surgeon K. Appel made a window with a diameter of 2 mm in an artery in the underarm and sewed an opened vein onto this window.[6] As a result that section of the vein filled itself with arterial blood and dilated so that it could be accessed easily with a needle through the skin

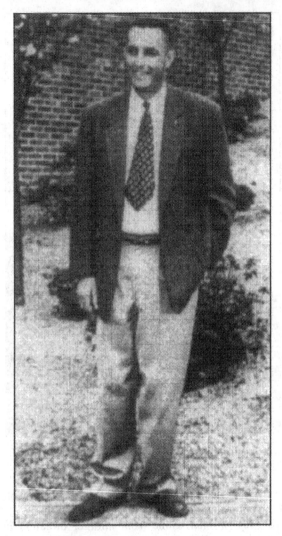

Figure 12.2 Clyde Shields, the first person to receive a Quinton–Scribner shunt.

for connection with the kidney. The blood was returned via a second needle that was pricked into the dilated vein downstream of the first one. Figure 12.4 gives a schematic view of the Cimino shunt.

12.2 HOME DIALYSIS

This technique made it possible to dialyse patients with chronic renal disease repeatedly, but then a new problem arose: every dialysis required a hospital

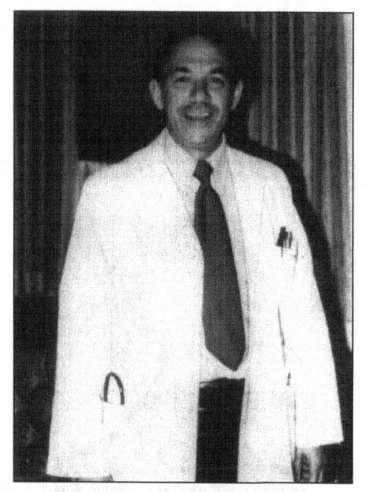

Figure 12.3   James Cimino, MD; the shunt he developed made it easier again for a patient to be dialysed repeatedly.

bed, and the costs kept on increasing. This impeded the extension of this mode of treatment.

In 1961 Shaldon in London (Figure 12.5) started a programme in which the patient assembled his own artificial kidney himself, connected himself to it and also stopped the dialysis himself; a nurse was within call only for help in case something went wrong.[7] One of the first patients using this technique is shown in Figure 12.6.

In Japan Nose started with home dialysis.[8] Scribner also developed home dialysis when the director of his hospital refused to keep more than 12 beds

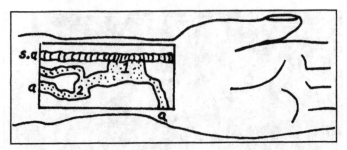

Figure 12.4 The so-called Cimino shunt. A window is cut in the radial artery and an opened vein is sewed onto it. Arterial blood is then obtainable by inserting a needle at (1). Blood that has passed the artificial kidney can be returned at (2).

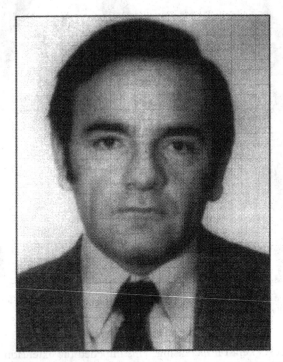

Figure 12.5 Stanley Shaldon, MD. He introduced home dialysis in the United Kingdom

free for dialysis patients. Merrill and his group in Boston also organized such a home dialysis; in 1964 Shaldon, Scribner and Merrill all reported on this development![9]

Scribner and his group used a kidney of the type developed by Kiil (to be described below). It had the advantage that no pump was needed to return the blood to the patient, but the treatment took 30 hours each week. Merrill and

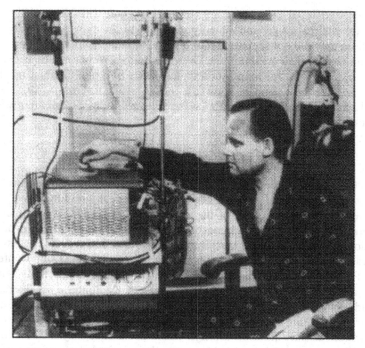

Figure 12.6   One of the first patients dialysing himself at home, as proposed by Shaldon.

his group used the 'twin-coil kidney'; its power was so high that only 12–14 hours in the daytime each week were required for dialysis – but that did require the use of a pump.

Meanwhile industrially produced kidneys were fitted with ever more automatic safety devices, and hence became ever more expensive. This was a thorn in Kolff's flesh. His standpoint was that many of these safety devices were superfluous provided the patient had been adequately trained. His favourite argument was that he believed in the motto of the first Volkswagen cars: 'What is not there cannot go wrong.' Experiments together with his eldest son (also a medical doctor) showed that the 'special bath' for the twin-coil kidney could be replaced very well by a simple washing machine that kept the water in motion. Together with his co-worker Dr Sat Nakamoto he succeeded in sending 28 patients home in 1966 with all the essential equipment, dialysing material and salts for the bath water enough for two months of dialysis at home, for a total sum of $263 (in comparison, when Kolff mentioned this in 1996 the annual costs of dialysis for a patient were $15 000–$25 000).[10] All went well until one day he was visited by the lawyer of the manufacturer of the washing machines, the Maytag Company. He told Kolff that his firm had noticed that Kolff bought their washing machines for this purpose – and that was something they objected to. If one day something went wrong with such a dialysis at home the patient would undoubtedly sue the firm for damages, and that was something they did not cherish. Hence the firm forbade Kolff from that moment on from buying their washing machines for dialysis. Was that the end of the cheap solution? Not for long. Another co-worker of Kolff, Stephen Jacobson, found that the nose-cone of a certain rocket, available from a dump store, would serve very well as the bath for the twin-coil kidney – and that was the origin of the 'nose-cone kidney'.

12.3   RENAL TRANSPLANTATION

While this was going on more knowledge was gained concerning organ transplantation. Rejection of a donor organ could often be prevented by a better study of the immune system of the donor and of the possible recipient. In addition it was found that adrenocortical hormones may be used to prevent rejection. In the early 1960s Merrill and Murray, in Boston, had success with the transplantation of kidneys into chronic renal patients. Kolff wanted to enter this road too, but the direction of the Cleveland Clinic flatly refused. That did not prevent Kolff from letting the surgeon Dr Poutasse rapidly remove the kidneys from six patients who were already on dialysis, and immediately after transplant into each of them the kidney of a relative. The reason for the removal of the patients' own kidneys was the fear that they would transmit the renal disease to the donor kidney. On the last Saturday morning clinical conference before the summer holidays Kolff could invite the six patients to take a seat on the platform – all blatantly well! That was the day when the renal transplantation programme was adopted in the Cleveland Clinic.[10]

Kolff and Nakamoto now continued by using the kidneys of deceased patients for transplantation – something that had gone out of use. When such a kidney is removed long after death renal cells may die. To counter this Kolff and Nakamoto treated the recipient of such a kidney with dialysis until the donor kidney had recovered: in one patient this took 120 days![10]

12.4   THE 1972 LEGAL REGULATION FOR REIMBURSEMENT

The number of dialyses increased in the 1960s as it became clear that this mode of treatment was effective. Because there were no financial means to treat all renal patients many hospitals installed selection committees that had to decide which patients would, and which patients would not, be treated. The task of these so-called 'Life-and-death' committees fortunately disappeared in 1972. The American Congress decided in that year, in connection with the law on 'Medicare', that the final stage of chronic renal disease was one of the financial catastrophes in the field of medicine: that meant that 80% of the costs would be paid by the Public Health Service (the Ministry of Public Health) for all patients covered by Social Security.

This legislation had enormous consequences. Many nephrologists who until then had not bothered with dialysis now found it to be financially interesting. It also provided the means to start new divisions for renal disease.

On the other hand it diminished the demand for simple, cheap apparatus in which the patient himself has to fulfil an active role. This legislation also inhibited the development of home dialysis in the United States. Scribner pointed out that when the legislation had been in effect for five years the number of patients on dialysis had risen to more than 30000, and that the costs were almost $1 billion; the percentage of renal patients on home dialysis had sunk from 41% in 1973 to less than 15% in 1977. This movement from home dialysis to dialysis in a clinic cost the American taxpayer another $150 million on top of the $1 billion in 1976.[11]

The forecast for 1979 was that the number of patients on dialysis in the United States would rise to a maximum of 60000, and that the costs would be about $2 billion in 1985. In reality the annual costs were between $8 billion and $9 billion in 1996. Is that realistic? Some persons in the United States started to ask. It meant that the community had to pay for this. It showed, according to Scribner, that we are entering the final stage of the era of unlimited growth of expensive medical technology – as clear as the signal of the oil crisis of 1973 that the end had come of the unlimited growth of the use of oil in the western community. The oil crisis showed, according to Scribner, that a democratic system is not able to set priorities in a crisis situation.

Does the development of dialysis and other costly medical techniques menace the free enterprise of the doctor such as practised especially in the United States? Scribner drew attention to the 'by-pass' operations on the coronaries that cost the American taxpayer at that time almost $2 billion per year, while at the same time doubt has arisen as to their significance for good health. The suspicion arose that this growth was directed more by free enterprise than by medical efficiency – in view of the fact that this operation is carried out on 28 patients per 100000 inhabitants in the United States, against 2.1 patients per 100000 inhabitants in Western Europe.[11]

Fortunately the efficiency of dialysis is not a matter for discussion from a medical point of view. However, Scribner called on his readers not to sit around in the present situation but to keep an eye on the possibilities of improving the cost–benefit ratio. How can we practise our responsibility towards the patients and at the same time lower the costs for the community of this still-expensive form of treatment.

Kolff referred to yet another case in which this financial regulation has an inhibitory effect. The pump that is usually employed in artificial kidneys and heart–lung machines for returning the blood to the patient shaves minute particles from the tube, which arrive in the patient with the returning blood – also in the cerebral vessels. Maybe they contribute to the changes that are often observed in the months following an open-heart operation (not in the case of dialysis: in this case the blood flow is at the most one-tenth of that in an open-heart operation). An improvement of that pump was developed in Kolff's laboratory – but neither industry nor the National Institutes of Public Health displayed any interest in this.

As stated above, the treatment of chronic renal patients cost the Department of Public Health in the United States $8 billion to $9 billion in 1996; the amount the National Institutes of Public Health devote each year to research on better and cheaper equipment for dialysis is no more than approximately 0.3% of this.[10]

12.5 THE TECHNICAL EVOLUTION OF THE ARTIFICIAL KIDNEY

Meanwhile the technical evolution of the kidney continued, also after the development of the 'twin-coil kidney' in 1955. Drukker gave an extensive review.[12] Roughly speaking, the original rotating kidney developed by Kolff has been succeeded by three types of non-rotating machines:

1. Kidneys using cellophane tube such as the twin-coil kidney of Kolff and Watschinger.
2. Kidneys using sheets of cellophane, such as the kidney of Skeggs and Leonards: the parallel-flow kidney.
3. Kidneys in which the blood flows through a large number of plastic capillaries surrounded by rinsing fluid: the capillary kidney or hollow-fibre kidney.

Contributions to the development of type 1 were made by Von Garrelts in Denmark, Michielsen in Belgium and Hoeltzenbein in Germany.[13] Kiil in Norway developed type 2 (see Figure 12.7), the parallel-flow kidney, into an apparatus that lent itself to mass production. The finding of Hoeltzenbein, in which the direction of flow of the rinsing fluid along the dialysing membrane was improved, has been applied in kidneys of type 1 and type 2.

Type 3 was developed by Stewart (see Figure 12.8): as a clinical chemist he had to deal with acute intoxications due to drug overdoses. He considered that he could make use of a principle that Mahon had applied in the purification of water: making fluid flow through hollow fibres with an internal diameter of 0.2 mm surrounded by another fluid. He set himself the task of developing a kidney with the same capacity as the twin-coil kidney.[14] His capillary kidney, with 11 000 capillaries, was first used on a patient in 1967. The whole apparatus is a cylinder with a length of about 20 cm and a diameter of about 10 cm; it is the type that is gradually gaining ground at the cost of the other two types (see Figure 12.9).

For the rest the capacities of the three types are very similar: the parallel-flow kidney and the capillary kidney have the advantage that they do not need a pump. The capillary kidney is the smallest of the three. Cellophane as the material for the dialysing surface is being replaced in all three types by cuprammonium cellulose or cuprophan, a synthetic derivative of cellulose facilitating

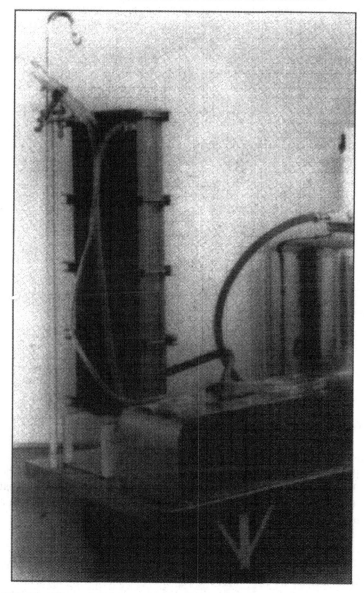

Figure 12.7   The Kiil parallel-plate dialyser with delivery system.

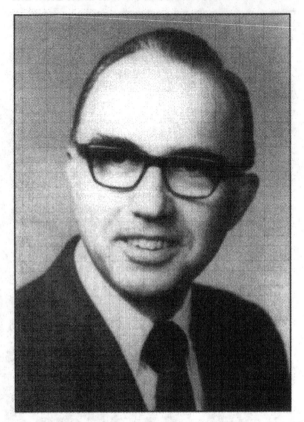

Figure 12.8   Richard Stewart, MD. He developed the hollow-fibre kidney.

a more rapid exchange of compounds between blood and rinsing fluid. Later on, still other synthetic materials came into use as a dialysing membrane.

All these developments contributed to an increase in the number of patients in the United States for whom some kind of dialysis was applied from about 1000 in 1967 to about 5000 three years later.[15]

12.6   DOES THE CLINICIAN MAKE AN EFFECTIVE USE OF WHAT IS TECHNICALLY AVAILABLE?

To his deep regret Scribner had to say 'No' to this question in 1996.[16] Nose had already remarked, before him, that the average survival time of chronic renal patients treated with dialysis in Japan was longer than in the United States.[17]

Why is that? Scribner mentions as the first cause that the duration of a dialysis in the United States is often too short. This is being facilitated in the

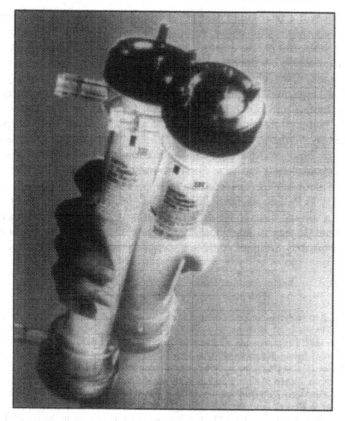

Figure 12.9 A hollow-fibre kidney with hollow fibres of cuprammonium cellulose or cuprophan. The total area of the fibres permitting dialysis is 1.6 square metres; the total length of this apparatus is only 25 cm.

commercial dialysis centres, as profits increase when as many patients as possible are being treated each week by as few members of medical personnel as possible. Bleyer reported at a meeting in 1995 that, in Australia, one dialysis on average was missed or stopped too soon per four patients per period of 4 months, whereas this figure was zero for Japan but five in the United States![18]

A second factor, according to Scribner, is the failure to lower the blood pressure sufficiently in patients with hypertension undergoing dialysis. The disastrous influence of hypertension (and smoking!) on the probability of survival of renal patients was described at the end of the 1970s. In 1992 B. Charra and his group, in France, showed that, with their dialysis technique, which at first sight appeared to be rather inefficient because a dialysis took many hours, good control of the patient's blood pressure was attainable, and with that a remarkably high probability of survival of their patients.[19]

Fortunately Scribner could also point to some successes. Patient number 5 in his group, who came under treatment in 1960, reached his 34th year of dialysis in 1995. In 1963 Scribner's group consented to treat an English medical student temporarily; in the next 30 years this student developed into a famous dermatologist at the University of London. He need not dialyse any longer, for in 1991 he received a donor kidney. In 1971 he described his experience as a patient, having undergone more than 1000 dialyses.[20]

A third factor decreasing the chances of survival of chronic renal patients, mentioned by Scribner, is the greater chance of acquiring another disease as they become older, and the high chance of already having a disease when they become chronic renal patients. Scribner mentions diabetes, cardiac disease, AIDS and drug use in this respect. The group of I. H. Khan in Scotland confirmed this.[21] 'Let us never forget', said Scribner, 'that a chronic renal disease is a *chronic* disease: let us get information from rehabilitation doctors and rheumatologists to learn techniques that bring success in chronic treatment.' Fortunately Scribner could see some developments in this direction.

NOTES

1. Gokal R. Replacement therapy by dialysis. In: Weatherall DJ, Ledingham JGG, Warrell DA,eds. *Oxford Textbook of Medicine*, 3rd edn. Oxford: Oxford University Press, 1996; vol. 3, pp. 3306–3312. The percentage of all renal patients making use of peritoneal dialysis varies very widely, from 5% in Japan to 90% in Mexico! Jacobs C, Kjellstrand CM, Koch KM and Winchester JF also estimated in 1996 the total number of people all over the world who are dependent on dialysis at more than half a million: see the 4th edition of the book *Replacement of Renal Function by Dialysis*, for which they formed the editorial board. It was published in Dordrecht by Kluwer Academic Publishers, 1996.
2. Teschan PE, Baxter CR, O'Brien TF *et al.* Prophylactic hemodialysis in the treatment of acute renal failure. *Annals of Internal Medicine* 1960; 53: 922–1016 (cited by McBride, see note 15, below).
3. Scribner BH, Dillard DH, Quinton WE. Cannulation of blood vessels for prolonged hemodialysis. *Transactions of the American Society for Artificial Internal Organs* 1960; 6: 104 (cited by Zenker W. *Die Entwicklungsgeschichte der extrakorporalen Hämodialyse von den Anfängen bis zur Routinetherapie in der Inneren Medizin*. Dortmund: Volker Keller, 1994).
4. Quinton WE, Dillard DH, Colle JJ, Scribner BH. Possible improvements in the technique of long-term cannulation of blood vessels. *Transactions of the American Society for Artificial Internal Organs* 1961; 7: 60 (cited by Zenker, see note 3, above). See also: Hegstrom RM, Quinton WE, Dillard DH, Cole JJ, Scribner BH. Two years experience with periodic hemodialysis in the treatment of uremia. *Transactions of the American Society for Artificial Internal Organs* 1962; 8: 266 (cited by Zenker, see note 3, above, p. 199).
5. Brescia MJ, Cimino JE. Simple venipuncture for hemodialysis. *New England Journal of Medicine* 1962; 267: 608 (cited by Zenker, see note 3, above, p. 202).
6. Cimino JE. Discussion in *Transactions of the American Society for Artificial Internal Organs* 1966; 12: 227 (cited by McBride, see ntoe 15, below, p. 53). Cimino describes the anastomosis between an artery and a vein designed by the surgeon Kenneth Appel. Other co-workers were Reuben Aboody, Michael Brescia and Baruch Hurwick.
7. Shaldon S. New developments with artificial kidney. *British Medical Journal* 1963; 1: 1685–1686 (cited by McBride, see note 15, below, p. 61).

8. Nose Y. Discussion on home dialysis. *Transactions of the American Society for Artificial Internal Organs* 1965; 11: 15 (in Japan from 1961 on) (cited by Zenker, see note 3, above, p. 217).

9. Shaldon S. Working Conference on Chronic Dialysis, Seattle. Proceedings, University of Washington, 1964 (see McBride, note 15, below, p. 61). See also Shaldon S, Oakley J, Sewitt L, 18 month experience with a nurse chronic dialysis unit. *Proceedings European Dialysis and Transplant Association* 1964; 1: 233 (cited by Zenker, see note 3, above, p. 217).

10. Kolff WJ. Early thoughts and spin-offs of the artificial kidney. *Dialysis and Transplantation* 1996; 25: 7146. Dr Sat Nakamoto and Kolff sent 28 patients home with a four-coil kidney they could wind themselves, at home, with a polyethylene network of Hoeltzenbein. See also: Khastagir B, Erben J, Shimizu A, Rose F, Nose Y, Van Dura D, Kolff WJ. *Transactions of the American Society for Artificial Internal Organs* 1967; 13: 14–18. See also, on renal transplantation: Kolff WJ, Nakamoto S. The re-establishment of cadaver kidney transplantation. Early kidney transplantation at the Cleveland Clinic. In: Terasaki P, ed. *History of Transplantation: Thirty-Five Recollections* 1996; pp. 245–266.

11. Scribner BH. Foreword, in Drukker W, Parsons FM, Maher JF, eds. *Replacement of Renal Function by Dialysis*, 2nd edn. The Hague: Martinus Nijhoff, 1978, pp. vii–viii.

12. Drukker W. Haemodialysis: a historical review. In: Drukker W, Parsons FM, Maher JF, eds. *Replacement of Renal Function by Dialysis*. The Hague: Martinus Nijhoff, 1978, pp. 3–37.

13. Hoeltzenbein J. *Die künstliche Niere – Apparative und klinische Grundlagen der extrakorporalen Hämodialyse*. Stuttgart: ENKE Verlag, p. 73 (cited by Zenker, see note 3, above, p. 248).

14. Stewart RD. The capillary artificial kidney. In: Bailey GL, ed. *Hemodialysis: Principles and Practice*. New York: Academic Press, 1972, pp. 382–396 (cited by McBride, see note 15, below, p. 64).

15. McBride PT. *Genesis of the Artificial Kidney*. Baxter Healthcare Corporation, 1987, p. 60. For his 'Ultraflo-coil' Baxter inserted tubes of cuprophan gauze according to Hoeltzenbein in a twin-coil kidney, and used a pump according to Sarns.

16. Scribner BH. Foreword to the fourth edition. In: Jacobs C, Kjellstrand CM, Koch KM, Winchester JF, eds. *Replacement of Renal Function by Dialysis*, 4th edn. Dordrecht: Kluwer Academic Publishers, 1996, pp. v–vi

17. Nose Y. The well-being of hemodialysis patients. *Artificial Organs* 1995; 19: 1201 (cited by Kolff, see note 10, above).

18. Wheeler D. Nephrologists focus on quality of care for chronic failure. *Lancet* 1996; 348: 1370.

19. Charra B, Calemard E, Ruffet M, Chazot C, Terrat JC, Vanel T, Laurent G. Survival as an index of adequacy in dialysis. *Kidney Internatinal* 1992; 41: 286.

20. Eady RAJ. A patient's experience of over one thousand haemodialyses. *Proceedings, European Dialysis and Transplantation Association* 1971; 8: 50 (cited by Scribner, see note 16, above).

21. Khan IH, Catto RDG, Edward N, Fleming LW, Henderson IS, MacLeod AM. Influence of coexisting disease on survival on renal-replacement therapy. *Lancet* 1993; 341: 415–418.

RENAL DIALYSIS IN THE NETHERLANDS AND IN EUROPE

13.1 RENAL DIALYSIS IN THE NETHERLANDS

Kolff's departure to Cleveland in 1950 caused a standstill in the development of dialysis in the Netherlands. The more so because Professor Borst at the University of Amsterdam preferred a low-protein, high-carbohydrate and fat diet for the treatment of renal patients. In addition he considered the risk of damage to the red blood cells by dialysis to be too high. The rotating kidney which Kolff had sent to Professor Borst's clinic in the University Hospital in Amsterdam was hence left unemployed.

However, dialysis was continued in Rotterdam. Dr Twiss, who had worked with Kolff in Kampen, organized a centre for dialysis in the Clara Hospital using the Alwall type of cellophane tubing artificial kidney. He attracted a number of young internists, and out of this arose the Dialysis Group Netherlands.

In 1959 the internist Dr W. Drukker succeeded in reintroducing dialysis in Amsterdam. In 1963 he developed the first programme in the Netherlands for chronic renal patients. Following the example of the American Society for Artificial Internal Organs, founded in 1954, he stimulated the foundation of the first European organization in this field in 1964: the European Dialysis and Transplantation Association (EDTA). It held its first international congress in Amsterdam in the same year. Later this organization became the European Renal Association. The annual meetings of this organization became an excellent forum for the exchange of information, the more so because almost 95% of all European dialysis centres took part.

In 1966 Drukker organized a data bank for dialysis and one for organ transplantation; later they were combined.

At that time the Netherlands had far too few dialysis centres for the treatment of chronic patients. For this problem too Drukker found a solution: together with the registered accountant Vogel, and with his friends, he started an organization to collect funds for more centres: the Netherlands Kidney Foundation, founded on 18 May 1967. When the Kiwanis Service Club of Amsterdam heard of the existence of the Kidney Foundation it started the Association in Support of the Kidney Foundation, in order to make it easier to collect money for the treatment of renal patients. This association gained extra attention at that time, because the first renal transplantation was carried out in Leiden in that year. Holidays for renal patients were organized for the first time in the same year.[1]

Together with Parsons and Maher, Drukker also edited the classical book on the replacement of renal function by dialysis with more than 40 contributions from experts all over the world.[2]

The 1991 report of the Health Council on dialysis and renal transplantation[3] and the 1997 paper by Huisman on dialysis in the elderly[4] give us the following picture of the treatment of chronic renal patients in the Netherlands.

In 1991 3201 chronic renal patients received some form of dialysis. More than 72% were dialysed in a centre, less than 4% dialysed at home and more than 24% had continuous ambulant peritoneal dialysis, or CAPD. This variant of the peritoneal dialysis which Kop had practised with Kolff in Kampen was introduced in 1972. It was applied by more than 30% of the renal patients in the provinces of North Holland and Gelderland, but only by about 10% of the patients in the provinces of Groningen, Friesland and Utrecht, where home dialysis had taken a much firmer root. As a matter of fact the percentage of patients using home dialysis decreased over the whole country and the percentage using CAPD rose. This is shown by the figures of 1 January 1994:[5] of the 3673 chronic renal patients who regularly used some form of dialysis 71% used an artificial kidney and 29% used CAPD. By the same date 3579 patients had received a donor kidney.

The average age of new dialysis patients rose from 43 years in 1975 to more than 57 years in 1994.[5] The percentage of patients aged 65 or older who were admitted to some form of dialysis rose from 23% in 1989 to 32% in 1994; this means that less than one-third of all chronic renal patients in that age group started dialysing.[4] The number of people aged 65 and over who start dialysis will probably continue to rise, the more so because this type of treatment brings much satisfaction to these patients, even more than to their doctors: regular visits to a dialysis centre bring social contacts that the elderly persons remaining at home often miss!

The annual number of renal transplantations rose in the Netherlands from 350 in 1985 to 400 in 1987, 1.5 times as rapidly as the number of patients starting dialysis. That indicates a rise to an annual number of 27 persons per million inhabitants – even so, we remain below the corresponding figure in the countries around us, where this figure is approximately 30 per million inhabitants. There is a long waiting list for renal transplantation in the Netherlands (1350 in 1990). We expected that the law on organ donation would lead to a shortening of that waiting list, but so far (in 2000) this has not come true.

The development of dialysis centres in the Netherlands also caused a large demand for assisting personnel. New professions arose, viz. the profession of dialysis nurse and of predialysis nurse. In 1995 the dialysis division of the hospital in Deventer (a town with a population of 69 000) received about 100 patients every week for haemodialysis and about 50 for CAPD. This involved

50 dialysis nurses (some part-time), two dieticians, two technicians, one assistant for courses, one predialysis nurse and five secretaries (some part-time).[6]

13.2 RENAL DIALYSIS IN EUROPE

Although Kolff had sent one of the four artificial kidneys he had at his disposal in 1945 to London, dialysis took a long time to get started in the United Kingdom. The leading internist, G. M. Bull, a man with great authority, was averse to such a machine, just like his colleague Borst in the Netherlands. He preferred to use a low-protein, high-calorie diet. The following summary is based on the full account given by Gurland et al.[7]

When dialysis got under way, nevertheless calculations showed that a steady increase in the number of dialysis patients would be possible only if an important fraction could be dialysed at home. Figures from 1976 indeed indicate that in the United Kingdom relatively more renal patients dialyse at home than the figures show elsewhere in Europe. The emphasis in other countries has been laid more on increasing the number of centres for dialysis.

Data from 1976 indicate how much dialysis has become accepted in Europe. An estimate indicated that 64 000 persons in the world owe their life to dialysis; 35% of them live in Europe, as many as in the United States. Of the remaining 30% two-thirds live in Japan. These data also show that confidence in dialysis has grown tremendously from the moment when repeated dialysis became possible thanks to the work of Scribner and of Cimino and their co-workers. Scribner formulated the criteria a patient had to meet for being admitted to a programme for repeated dialysis. If these criteria had been observed without change in 1976, 70% of these 64 000 patients would never have been admitted to such a programme! Especially in countries with at least two dialysis centres per million inhabitants the number of patients on some kind of dialysis increased enormously; this applies to, *inter alia*, the Netherlands, Belgium, Germany, Spain, Greece, Italy, France, Switzerland, Norway, Finland and Iceland.

Table 13.1 shows that the percentage of renal patients receiving a donor

Table 13.1 Percentages of chronic renal patients receiving a donor kidney in 1975

Country	Percentage receiving a donor kidney
Norway	73
Finland	60
Denmark	52
Sweden	47
Iceland	44
United Kingdom	36
Switzerland	35
United States	25

kidney was high in all Scandinavian countries. In the Netherlands 465 chronic renal patients received a donor kidney in 1991, or 13% of all chronic renal patients.[3]

Changes in the type of artificial kidney used in Europe between 1982 and 1992 are shown in Table 13.2.[8]

13.3   RENAL DIALYSIS IN THE HOLIDAYS

As the development of equipment for dialysis made it more and more possible for chronic renal patients to lead a life that did not differ too much from a normal one, the desire grew stronger to also include the possibilities of a holiday. The use of a large caravan was one of the first of these in the United States, where the use of such large vehicles is much older than in Europe. Of course this implied that the patient, or members of his or her family, should be able to handle the dialysing machine, and that electric power, clean water and a telephone were available.

Of course it did not stop there. The patients acquired a taste for it and wanted more and more. One of them wished to go rafting through the Grand Canyon. Would that really be impossible? But why, after all? Suppose that, between the days on the raft, there were a day in a camp where the patient could dialyse? There would have to be a van to bring supplies to the camp, and that van could just as well bring an artificial kidney. And then, what about going to Hawaii and lying on the beach with a dialysing machine; why not?

And so a travel organization, 'Dialysis in Wonderland', arose in the United States under the leadership of John Warners.[9]

The possibilities for spending holidays in this way were increased enormously in theory by the development of the 'Wearable Artificial Kidney', or WAK, by Stephen Jacobsen;[10] before that he had developed the 'nose-cone kidney'. Mountaineering with pauses for dialysing with a WAK appeared to become possible. The WAK could be so compact because it was a kind of capillary tube kidney with adsorbing filters, developed when space travel brought the need to recycle waste water – including urine – to drinking water! Whenever he had a chance Kolff stimulated its application, as shown for example in Figure 13.1.

It was one of the deep disappointments of Kolff that he failed to find a producer for the WAK, after use of 20 specimens had shown what this apparatus

Table 13.2   Type of artificial kidney used in Europe in 1982 and 1992 (in percentages)

Type of kidney	1982	1992
Cellophane tube	7	0
Parallel flow	>37	<7
Capillary tube	52	>93

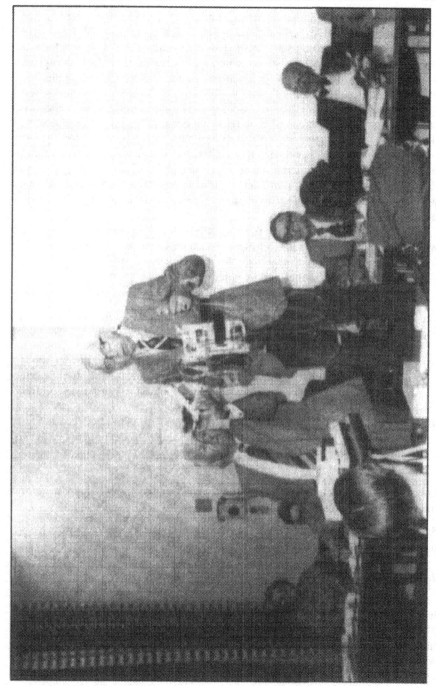

Figure 13.1 Standing on a chair Kolff demonstrates the wearable artificial kidney at a workshop of the Kidney Foundation in Utrecht.

could mean for a chronic renal patient. To make the production worthwhile it would have to be sold for a price three times as high as the cost of manufacture, and then the WAK would cost more than an ordinary dialysing machine as used in the dialysis centres. This was regrettable the more because a holiday with 'Dialysis in Wonderland' could bring patients unforgettable memories, and so strengthen their feeling that they could steer their life's course themselves.

One of these patients asked her doctor after such a holiday trip: 'Doctor, can't you ask your colleague who dialysed me during that trip exactly what he did? I felt so much better after a dialysis on that trip than when you dialyse me at home.' 'Madam', her doctor replied, 'He did exactly what I had told him before you left, but the difference is in you yourself: you enjoyed your trip and therefore you took a much more active view on life.' Her doctor reported this when he spoke at a meeting on dialysis held in Salt Lake City in 1986 in honour of Kolff's 75th birthday.

In Europe too the desire grew to make it possible to break the daily routine with a holiday trip. It was part of the desire to make life as normal as possible for such patients. Another argument for enabling renal patients to travel is that travelling is an essential part of some professions.

Davison mentions seven ways for enabling kidney patients to travel:[11]

1. Prolonging the interval between successive dialyses up to five days.
2. Choice of a holiday resort near home, and returning home for the next dialysis.
3. Finding a dialysis centre near the desired holiday resort. The address books of the European Dialysis and Transplant Association, and the Seattle Artificial Kidney Supply Company (SAKSCO) mention 541 dialysis centres in 41 countries offering facilities for this purpose.
4. Temporary removal of the whole dialysis centre to a holiday resort. This has been done, e.g., in Belgium, offering a holiday to 22 patients with 50 members of their families! Of course this option demands a lot of organization.

Options 5 to 7 demand much more activity from the individual patient or members of the family:

5. Dialysis with the patient's own equipment in a hotel room.
6. Dialysis in a caravan with the patient's own equipment (this option has been described above as the starting point for 'Dialysis in Wonderland').
7. Holidays with a WAK. Something for the future?

As mentioned above, Kolff did not succeed in realizing this idea. However, it is fascinating to reflect whether this may not become possible in the future. Stewart developed his capillary kidney from apparatus designed to purify water, fulfilling a requirement induced by the wish to travel in space. Pure drinking water is becoming a scarce commodity all over the world. Hence we may expect that efforts are being made all over the world to develop simpler and cheaper ways to purify water. If a side-product of this were a small portable apparatus with which blood could be purified without bacterial or viral contamination, such a portable kidney might come within the reach of very many chronic renal patients after all.

That would be of great significance. The wall separating a chronic renal patient from everyday life crumbles further when the patient can go on holiday – but only having a small wearable kidney at his or her disposal makes the bearer forget that he or she is a patient.

NOTES

1. These data are taken from the contribution of Jos Arnoudse to the book published in 1992 on the 15th anniversary of the Netherlands association of renal patients, LVD.
2. Drukker W, Parsons FM, Maher JF, eds. *Replacement of Renal Function by Dialysis*, 2nd edn. The Hague: Martinus Nijhoff, 1979.
3. Koomans HA, Blankestein PJ. Report of the Health Council on dialysis and renal transplantation. *Nederlands Tijdschrift voor Geneeskunde* 1993; 137:748–749.
4. Huisman RM. Dialysis in the old. *Nederlands Tijdschrift voor Geneeskunde* 1997; 141: 229–233.
5. TNO Prevention and Health. Investing in the prevention of renal disease: an investment in the future. Note to the Nierstichting Nederland (Netherlands Renal Foundation). *DIA*, 1994; 24: December, p. 9.
6. See *DIA*, 1995; 25: June, p. 12.
7. Gurland HJ, Wing AJ, Jacobs C, Brunner F. Comparative review between dialysis and transplantation. In: Drukker W, Parsons FM, Maher JF, eds. *Replacement of Renal Function by Dialysis*, 2nd edn. The Hague: Martinus Nijhoff, 1979, pp. 663–684.
8. Hoenich NA, Woffindin C, Ronco C. Haemodialysers and associated devices. In: Jacobs C, Kjellstrand CM, Koch KM, Winchester JF, eds. *Replacement of Renal Function by Dialysis*, 4th edn. Dordrecht: Kluwer, 1996, pp. 188–230.
9. See the NOS television programme 'Markant' devoted to Kolff, February 1989.
10. Kolff WJ. The future of dialysis. In: Drukker W, Parsons FM, Maher JF, eds. *Replacement of Renal Function by Dialysis*, 2nd edn. The Hague: Martinus Nijhoff, 1979, pp. 702–710. See also: Stephen RL, Jacobsen SC, Atkin-Thor E, Kolff WJ. Portable wearable artificial kidney (WAK) – initial evaluation. *Proceedings, European Dialysis and Transplant Association* 1975; 12: 511.
11. Davison AM. Holidays for dialysis patients. In: Drukker W, Parsons FM, Maher J, eds. *Replacement of Renal Function by Dialysis*, 2nd edn. The Hague: Martinus Nijhoff, 1989, pp. 482–485.

14

ON THE SHOULDERS OF KOLFF

When Isaac Newton declared that he could make great contributions to science because he stood on the shoulders of giants, science was an activity of single persons, so that Newton could name every one of them. Among the predecessors of Kolff we find a group of three persons, *viz.* Abel, Rowntree and Turner. The past half-century has seen an enormous growth of teamwork in the sciences. Therefore we run the risk of being incomplete when we want to mention those who have continued making new constructions based on Kolff's ideas. The more so because the composition of those teams changes all the time.

In addition the environment of those teams changes, sometimes producing as a byproduct something which fills a long-existing need for the group.

After Kolff had left the Cleveland Clinic the University of Utah provided him with more opportunities to work out his ideas. There he could give a shape to his ideas on a heart–lung machine, an artificial heart and a better twin-coil kidney. However, it characterizes him that he did not start an Institute for Renal Disease or for Cardiac Disease, but an Institute for Artificial Organs. 'Pim Kolff is that rare bird that has to settle down in more than one tree of knowledge to be satisfied, unfold his talents and follow his ideas' was the way Burton characterized him.[1] He succeeded in creating in his institute an atmosphere of expectation as long as something was being done or made. Although he had been trained neither as an engineer nor as a biochemist he quickly grasped the essentials of most proposals made to him – irrespective of whether the subject was a wearable artificial kidney or artificial muscles or an artificial eye. The next thing he did was to sketch a number of possible applications, then he went to work. The only thing he did not appreciate was hesitancy.

We shall not describe here the work on the artificial heart and on an artificial eye, but only the work designed to widen the range of solutions for chronic renal patients. The Netherlands Kidney Foundation recognized this by creating the annual award of the 'Kolff Medal' to the person who had distinguished himself or herself in the field of the treatment or the welfare of renal patients. Of course Kolff was the first person to receive one (see Figure 14.1).

In contrast with the idea of an implantable artificial heart Kolff saw no reason to go for an implantable artificial kidney. The three types of artificial kidney now available – the cellophane tube kidney, the parallel-flow kidney

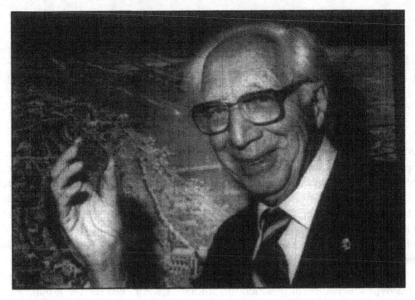

Figure 14.1 Kolff with the 'Kolff Medal', awarded by the Netherlands Kidney Foundation to persons who have rendered important services to renal patients.

and the capillary tube kidney – have sufficient capacity to let the patient work for a number of hours without being connected to it. Peritoneal lavage, also available as CAPD (or continuous ambulant peritoneal dialysis) is preferable to haemodialysis for some patients. Peritoneal lavage was also a target for the ingenuity of Kolff's co-workers. They developed the 'mouse': a hollow sack of Dacron the size of a finger, kept open inside by a cylindrical spring and with a rough outside. The sack opened into a smooth tube. The sack was fixed in the patient's abdominal wall in such a way that the tube opened into the peritoneal cavity. Entrance to the mouse was obtained with a needle through the skin.[2]

Some patients under treatment with peritoneal dialysis had diabetes and regularly injected insulin. The development of the mouse made someone ask whether this could not also be used for these injections. The result was the development of the 'SPAD', the subcutaneous peritoneal access device: a sack in the shape of a hollow mushroom that was implanted under the skin and was open to the peritoneal cavity.[3] This device for administering insulin proved to have two advantages over the traditional subcutaneous injection: (1) 80% of the insulin administered in this way reaches the liver directly via the portal vein; (2) less lipids are deposited in the walls of the arteries because less insulin circulates through the blood vessels.[4]

The energy with which Kolff kept on working on many different projects after his 75th birthday is hard to imagine. Someone asked Chase Petersen, the

President of the University of Utah, whether he could imagine what would happen if Kolff were no longer able to go on with his work: 'Then we'll just replace the worn parts with the artificial organs he has made himself and then the work will just go on', was his reply.[5]

NOTES

1. Burton BT. Notes of a Kolff-watcher. *Nephron* 1984; 36: 159–160.
2. Kablitz C, Kessler T, Dew PA, Stephen RL, Kolff WJ. Subcutaneous peritoneal catheter: 2½ years experience. *Artificial Organs* 1979; 3: 210–214.
3. Kablitz C, Stephen RL, Harrow JC, Nelson JA, Tyler FH, Hanover BK, Jacobsen SC. Subcutaneous peritoneal dialysis access device used for intraperitoneal insulin treatment of non-uraemic diabetic patients. Proceedings, Second International Symposium in Peritoneal Dialysis, Berlin, 1981, pp. 170–172.
4. Bell JI, Hockaday TDR. Diabetes mellitus. In: Weatherall DJ, Ledingham JGG, Warrell DA, eds. *Oxford Textbook of Medicine*, 3rd edn. Oxford: Oxford University Press, 1996, vol. II: p. 1478.
5. NOS television programme, 'Markant', transmitted in February 1989.

15

HAS KOLFF REACHED HIS GOAL?

When Kolff was struck by the fate of a young man dying of chronic nephritis in 1938 he set himself the goal of developing a dialysing apparatus which could tide a renal patient over a temporary decrease of renal function, or at least attain a temporary improvement.

Apart from temporary improvements in the first 16 patients this goal was achieved very clearly in the case of patient 17, who recovered completely from her hepatorenal syndrome. In December 1946 a man of 23 years recovered after an accidental intoxication with bichloride of mercury. Bywaters reported the recovery of a patient with oliguria after an explosion (crush syndrome?).[1]

The development of the rotating artificial kidney was followed by the development of other apparatus, and of new methods for treating renal patients. Peritoneal dialysis enabled Kolff and Kop to discharge six out of 21 patients with an adequate renal function.

Suppose that the young man with chronic nephritis and the first 15 patients that Kolff treated between 1943 and 1944 came under treatment today; what would their fate be?

The young man from Groningen and patient number 1 from Kampen had chronic nephritis. They would now probably dialyse regularly with a capillary tube kidney or apply peritoneal lavage while waiting for a donor kidney.

Patient number 2 had tuberculosis of the kidneys and the bladder. The chemotherapy he would receive nowadays did not exist then. Depending on the degree of loss of function he would probably be either discharged from treatment or dialyse until he could get a donor kidney.

Patient number 4 had cancer of the bladder; patient number 9 renal cancer. If there were any chance of success they would get chemotherapy now and probably dialyse while waiting for a donor kidney.

Patients number 12 and 15 had an intoxication with bichloride of mercury. That can be treated now with a specific antidote, dimercaprol. In their case, too, further treatment would depend on the results. The most likely outcomes would now be discharge in good health or dialyse until a donor kidney had become available.

The renal failure of patients number 5 and 14 started after an operation: how this came about is not clear.

The renal function of patients numbers 3, 6, 11 and 13 deteriorated as a result of an acute nephritis. The high blood potassium level of patient number 3 would nowadays be detected at a much earlier stage, so that it could be taken into account in the dialysis. Patient number 6 had nephritis as a complication of scarlet fever. Her pneumonia would now have been treated with antibiotics. These four patients would now probably have been tided over their acute nephritis. Unless their kidneys had been damaged too much they would be discharged in good health.

The same, in effect, obtains for patient number 8 who had a nephritis with a more protracted course.

We saw that patient number 10 was the only one of this series of 15 who was discharged in good health in 1944.

What about patient number 7, the man whose right kidney was removed because of a staphylococcal infection and who proved to have no functioning left kidney? In the first place his staphylococcal infection would now be fought with antibiotics. The absence of a functioning left kidney would probably be discovered at an earlier stage now, and his treatment would be focused on supporting the infected right kidney with a diet and with dialysis; removal of the inflamed right kidney would probably not be done.

In short, the development of better tools for fighting bacterial infection, including tuberculosis, better tools for fighting mercurial intoxication and better anticancer drugs would now make it easier to overcome their renal failure with dialysis. The target that Kolff set himself in 1938 has come within reach in recent decades; it has in fact been reached by countless patients all over the world.

Charles Darwin's phrase, 'Seeing what everyone sees – thinking what no-one has thought', has in fact been practised by Kolff – although Kolff's interest is focused so much on doing things that I doubt whether he has ever read Darwin's reflection. It is typical for Kolff that he saw possibilities for use in objects developed for quite a different purpose – the development of the twin-coil kidney is a typical example.

The targets Kolff set himself increased with time. His public lecture after his appointment as Reader at the University of Leiden was entitled 'Life without heart and kidneys'; he painted a picture of a person whose malfunctioning heart and kidneys had been replaced by an artificial heart and artificial kidneys, small enough to be carried in a backpack while the person was doing his work. Has this science fiction been realized?

We saw that the wearable artificial kidney was a medical success but an economic failure in spite of all the energy of Kolff and his co-workers. Kolff kept on working on an artificial heart at the University of Utah long after his 75th birthday. His hearts prolong the life of many patients waiting for a donor heart.

His division of artificial organs and his Institute for Biomedical Technique have widened the limits of the meaning of 'artificial organ' far beyond imagination in the past. When he was a child only the words 'artificial arm' or 'artificial leg' indicated something one could form a mental picture of. An artificial or glass eye was something that could be seen, but that could not itself see. Nowadays not only artificial kidneys but also artificial hearts, artificial muscles, an artificial hand, an artificial eye enabling the wearer to really see, have all become real.

All this did not just happen. Kolff has not been spared jealousy and criticism. The application of the artificial heart in Barney Clark in 1982 led to fierce criticism and fighting of that criticism in the United States. Kolff did not take part in that battle.

> The less attention one pays to such criticism, the better. In fact I hardly ever react, with very few exceptions. Many years ago the medical press published papers saying that the artificial kidney was not really necessary. I did not react. If I had done so I would now have had many enemies and I would probably have turned into a paranoid fighter. Just let it go. My standpoint has not changed, I think I have taken it over from my father. It is a very simple philosophy: if you can help some people you must do so – if you cannot help them you must help them end their lives with as little pain as possible.[2]

In May 1991 the Netherlands Dialysis Group held a two-day symposium in Kampen to commemorate the beginning of Kolff's career as an 'organ maker' in the town hospital 50 years ago. On that occasion he was interviewed by Jean-Paul Berting, a journalist who had dialysed himself for some years and who had undergone two kidney transplantations. This interview has been published in DIA, 1991, number 2, the magazine of the Netherlands Kidney Foundation and the Association of Friends of the Netherlands Kidney Foundation. At the end of this interview Berting asked Kolff whether he had also received recognition from the kidney patients, in addition to the countless decorations he had received in the medical world. Kolff's answer was typical for his permanent willingness to help other persons and for his sober-mindedness:

> As regards my own patients I have the most happy experience in that respect. But if you ask whether the average dialysis patient knows that W. J. Kolff has had something to do with the artificial kidney: no, they do not know about it.
>
> There are some dialysis centres that have been given my name. Three weeks ago I was in one of them. I opened the door for an old lady in a wheelchair and helped her get into the elevator. She asked me who I was and I mentioned my name. Then she said: 'Do you know anything about dialysis?'! In my own building!
>
> I have got used to that. Never mind. You know that there are a quarter of a million people in the world dependent upon dialysis.

NOTE

1. Bywaters EGL in: Kolff WJ with the cooperation of J. van Noordwijk, P. S. M. Kop, N. K. M. de Leeuw and A. M. Joekes. *New Ways of Treating Uraemia.* London: J & A Churchill, 1947; page 38.
2. Burton BT. Notes of a Kolff-watcher. *Nephron* 1984; 36: 159–160.

16

A NEW LIFE FOR OLD DIALYSERS

The hospital 'De Engelenbergstichting' in Kampen continued to function until 1994, when the Ministry of Public Health adopted a policy of closing down 'small hospitals', that is hospitals with less than 200 beds, and concentrating hospital service in large hospitals. An outpatient clinic was opened adjacent to the hospital grounds in Kampen, but patients had to go to the nearby town of Zwolle for treatment in hospital.

An attempt to preserve the hospital building as a national monument because of its architectural value was made in 1996: it was one of the few intact buildings designed by the architect Willem Kromhout in the Dutch version of the 'Art Nouveau' or 'Jugendstil', but the town council of Kampen hesitated and eventually refrained from supporting this project.

In 1998 an old-age home in Kampen made plans for a new larger building and situated this in the hospital grounds, necessitating the demolition of the hospital building. When this became known a committee formed in Kampen to save the hospital building. Kolff had decided shortly before to revisit Kampen, and when he heard this alarming news he did all he could to stop these plans. He was received by the Minister of Public Health, Dr E. Borst: the cost of demolition would have to be paid by her ministry and she promised to contribute funds equal to the cost of demolition if the hospital building could be conserved to house a museum of artificial organs. Unfortunately a confirmation of this only reached Kampen the day after the town council of Kampen had decided 'with a bleeding heart' in July 1999 to demolish the hospital in order to facilitate the building of the old-age home.

On hearing of the minister's confirmation the committee to save the hospital contacted the local radio. The result was an interview with Kolff in an international radio programme three days later. This was also heard by a Dutch former kidney patient on holiday in the south of France, and he immediately donated a large sum of money to help save the hospital building! The committee to save the hospital submitted a request to the Minister of Education, Art and Sciences to grant the status of a national monument to the hospital building because of its architectural value: it was the only hospital building in the 'Art Nouveau' style by Willem Kromhout still in existence. Kolff organized a tour by the committee to Ingolstadt in Germany, where Professor Christa Habrich had won a similar fight to preserve the 18th-century building where the German Medical Museum was housed. Shortly after that experts from the Ministry of Education visited Kampen to see the hospital building and discuss the request to recognize it as a national monument. The enthusiasm of these experts contributed to make the aldermen of Kampen change their opinion about the hospital building. A decision to place a building on the list of national monuments can be taken only when the relevant municipal council submits a formal request to do so. When the procedure had reached this stage in Kampen, the aldermen advised the council to make such a request: the council did so in fact on 23 March 2000 by a unanimous vote. The official decision to grant the status of national monument is expected to be published in October 2000.

This development is of great importance for two subgroups of the human population. The unique hospital building in 'Art Nouveau' style will be a landmark for anyone interested in the development of architecture in the 20th century in Europe. For persons who use an artificial or a transplanted kidney it will be a unique experience to enter the building and see with their own eyes the rooms where the development started which made it possible to save their lives. These rooms are destined to be part of a museum of artificial organs, to be housed in an adjacent building that was used as a school in those days. Further material will be on site there – building bricks and mortar for the developments that opened up new hopes of life for people with failing kidneys, hearts, hands, eyes and ears – all over the world.

9 780792 367628